Dr. Nowzaradan's Diet Plan

The Scales Don't Lie, People Do! The Only 1200 kcal Diet from Dr. NOW to Lose Weight Fast. 30-Day Diet Plan + Simple and Healthy Recipes

Ramirez Sanchez

Summary

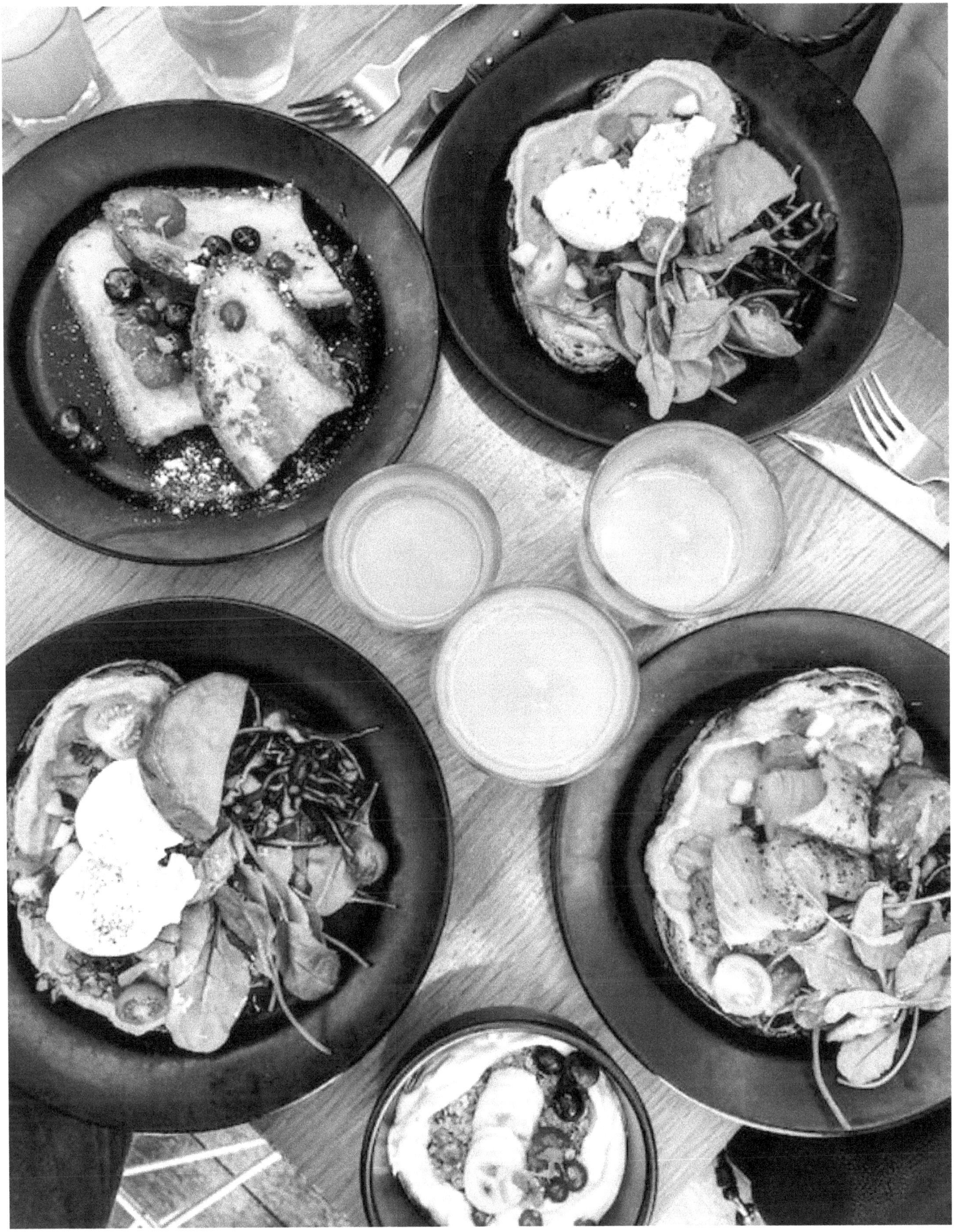

Foreword

Welcome to a journey that could change not only your weight, but also your outlook on health, nutrition and life itself. When you pick up this book, you may be at the beginning of a path that many before you have traveled with hope and a desire for profound change. Dr. Younan Nowzaradan, also known as Dr. Now, has inspired and helped thousands of people with his groundbreaking work in bariatric surgery. His approach, which goes far beyond the operating room, emphasizes the importance of a comprehensive lifestyle change that begins with a carefully designed diet.

This book is intended as a guide to help you understand and apply the principles and practices of Dr. Now's Diet Plan for Beginners. It is written for those who want to take the first step toward a healthier life, whether they choose to have surgery or simply embark on a more sustainable, healthier lifestyle.

Dr. Nowzaradan's diet plan may seem intimidating at first glance, especially because of its strict calorie restriction and list of "forbidden" foods. But behind this strictness lies a deeper truth about the way we eat, live and take care of our health. This plan is not just a diet; it is an invitation to re-evaluate and change your life.

In the following chapters, we'll explain the basics of Dr. Now's diet plan, provide practical tips and advice to get you started, and outline strategies for achieving long-term success. Whether you're looking to lose weight, improve your health or are just curious about how to change your eating habits, this book will give you the knowledge and tools you need to achieve your goals.

Our goal is for you to feel empowered to make positive changes in your life after reading this book. We want you to understand that weight loss and healthy eating are not just about numbers on a scale or strict diet plans, but about a holistic sense of well-being and the joy that comes with healthy living.

Join us on this journey. There will be challenges and obstacles, but the rewards - a healthier, happier you - are worth every step.

Introduction

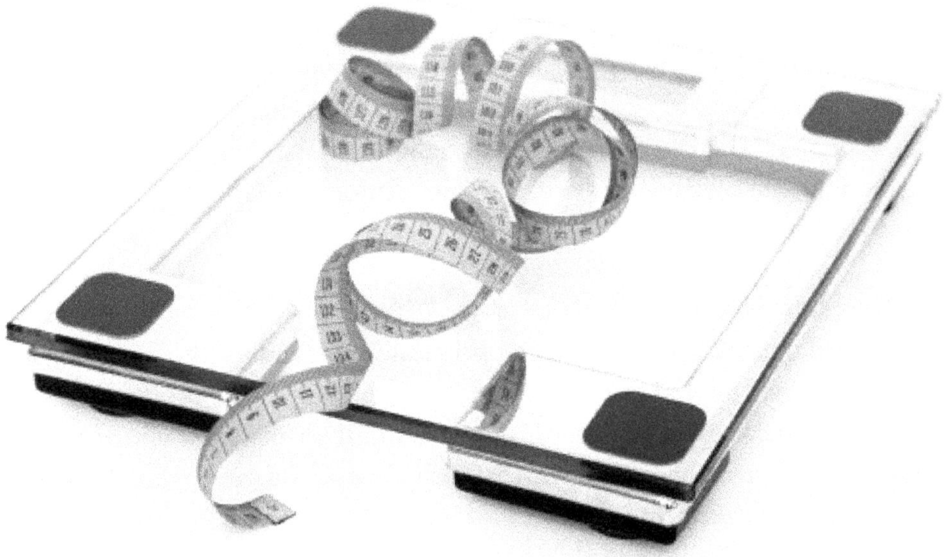

When talking about weight loss and transformation, it's impossible to pass over the work of Dr. Younan Nowzaradan - affectionately known as Dr. Now. His approach to weight loss has gained recognition not only in the medical community, but also among the general public through the popular television series "My 600-lb Life." But what exactly makes Dr. Now's approach so special, and why has he helped so many people change their lives?

Dr. Nowzaradan's philosophy is based on the premise that successful weight loss and maintaining a healthy lifestyle go far beyond surgical intervention. While bariatric surgery can be an important tool to save lives and address serious health issues, Dr. Now emphasizes the importance of nutrition, psychological support and sustainable lifestyle changes.

One of the key aspects of his approach is preparing patients for the profound changes they will experience after surgery. This begins with a strict diet designed to reduce weight before surgery, minimize the risk of complications and prepare patients for the necessary post-operative adjustments. Dr. Now's diet is not just a short-term solution; rather, it is the first step on the road to a new, healthier you.

Another key aspect of Dr. Now's approach is individualized care. Each patient is unique, with their own needs, challenges and goals. Dr. Now tailors his treatment and advice to individual circumstances, always with the goal of finding the best and safest route to weight loss. This customized approach not only helps patients to lose weight, but also to gain a new self-confidence and a new perspective on health and well-being. Dr. Nowzaradan also places great emphasis on providing psychological support to his patients. He understands that overweight and obesity often have deep-rooted emotional and psychological causes. Through conversation, therapeutic support and encouraging self-reflection, Dr. Now helps his patients overcome the emotional hurdles that stand in the way of successful weight loss.

In this book chapter, we will dive deeper into the fundamentals of Dr. Nowzaradan's diet and weight loss strategies. We will explore the principles behind the famous 1200 calorie diet, emphasize the importance of exercise and physical activity, and discuss the role of psychological support in the weight loss process. The goal is to give you a clear understanding of how Dr. Now's comprehensive approach can help you take the first steps toward a healthier, more fulfilling life.

Why this book is important for you

In a world where information about health and wellbeing is more abundant than ever before, it can be a real challenge to separate the signal from the noise. Dietary advice comes and goes, and what is hailed as the ultimate in nutritional science today may be considered outdated tomorrow. Amidst this confusing flood of information, Dr. Younan Nowzaradan's approach stands like a beacon of clarity and effectiveness. This book is your ticket to a world where weight loss is not just a temporary goal, but a permanent state of well-being and health. You may be wondering why this book in particular can make all the difference in your life. The answer lies in the simplicity and depth of Dr. Now's method. By applying the principles and strategies detailed in the following chapters, you will not only gain the tools to lose weight, but also the ability to fundamentally change your relationship with food.

This book is important for you because it:

1. **offers practical instructions:** Instead of vague advice, you'll get clear, practical steps you can implement immediately. From detailed nutrition plans to recipes specifically designed for the beginning of your journey, you'll be shown a path that is feasible and sustainable.
2. **Scientifically sound:** Every recommendation in this book is based on the latest nutritional science and Dr. Now's decades of experience in treating patients with extreme obesity. You can be sure that the advice you will find here is not only safe, but also effective.
3. **Psychological support:** Weight loss is not only a physical challenge, but also an emotional one. This book recognizes the psychological aspects of weight loss and offers strategies to deal with stress, emotional eating and loss of motivation.
4. **Inspired and motivated:** Through success stories of people who have followed Dr. Now's diet, you will be shown that change is possible. These stories serve as proof that no matter how hopeless your situation may seem, there is always a way forward.
5. **Designed for the long term:** This book lays the foundation for lasting change. You will learn how to maintain your new habits and keep a healthy weight in the long term.

Whether you're preparing for bariatric surgery or simply looking for a proven approach to weight loss, this book is an indispensable companion on your journey to a healthier you. It's not just about shedding pounds; it's about gaining a new life. A life where you feel energized, confident and above all healthy. Take the first step on this journey by turning the pages of this book.

Chapter 1: Understand the basics

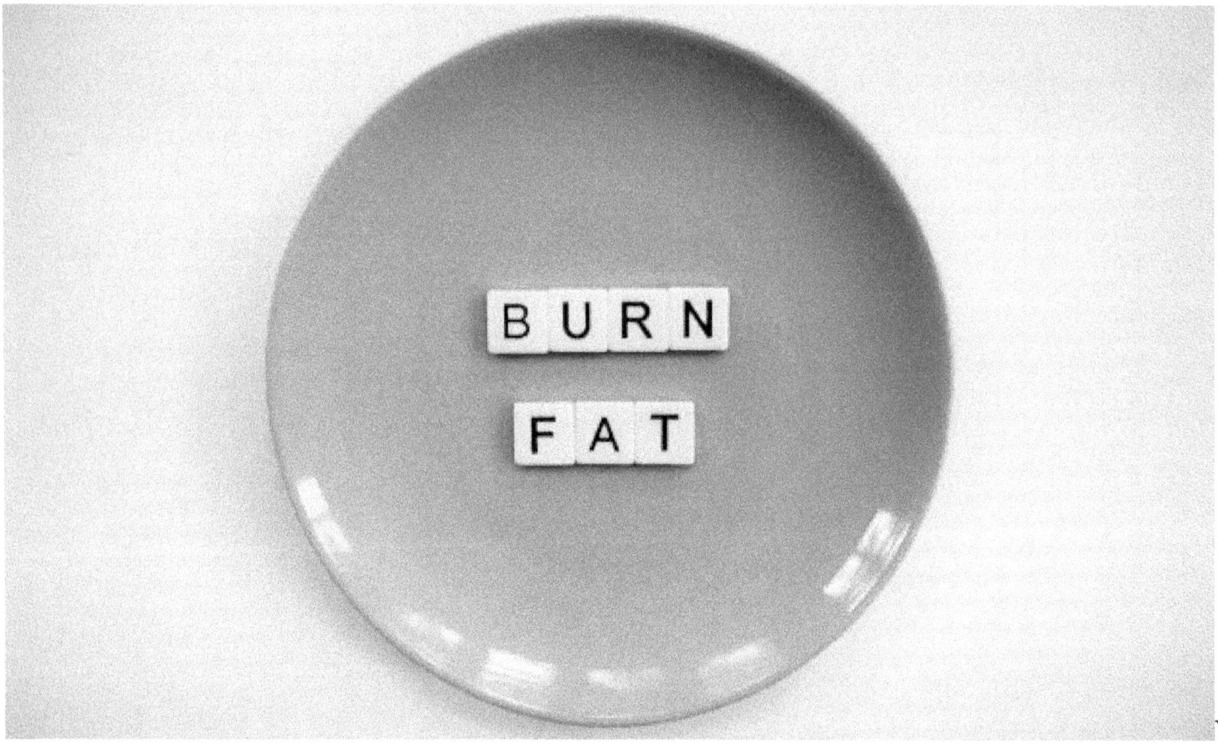

Welcome to the first chapter of your journey to a healthier self. Before we dive into the specific guidance and advice that will transform your body and mind, it's crucial to establish a solid foundation. Understanding the foundational principles upon which Dr. Nowzaradan's approach is based will not only strengthen your motivation, but also give you the tools to make informed decisions about your health.

Principle 1: The philosophy behind the plan

Dr. Younan Nowzaradan, known for his empathetic yet pragmatic approach to weight loss, sees the need for holistic change. His philosophy goes beyond just calorie counting and focuses on the wellbeing of the whole person. Weight loss, in his eyes, is not just a physical journey, but an emotional and psychological transformation.

Principle 2: The role of nutrition

One of the pillars of Dr. Now's approach is a balanced, nutrient-rich diet. Limiting yourself to 1200 calories a day may seem strict at first, but the key lies in the quality, not just the quantity, of the food you consume. This chapter will help you understand the importance of macro and micronutrients and how thoughtful food choices can nourish your body and promote weight loss.

Principle 2: The importance of calorie reduction

Calorie reduction is a key element of Dr. Now's diet plan, but it's about much more than simply counting calories. It's about developing a deep understanding of how different foods affect your body and learning how to make conscious choices that lead to lasting weight loss.

Principle 3: Adapt your lifestyle

Dr. Now emphasizes that lasting change can only be achieved through lifestyle adjustments. This chapter guides you through the first steps to reshaping your daily routines and habits to incorporate a healthy diet and regular exercise. You'll discover how small changes can lead to significant results over time.

Principle 4: The psychological component

A key component of success lies in overcoming psychological barriers. From dealing with emotional eating to overcoming motivation lows, this chapter covers the mental aspects of weight loss and offers strategies to face the challenges that arise along the way with strength and confidence.

Summary

The foundation for successful weight loss and healthy living is laid through a deep understanding of the basics. By understanding the philosophy, principles of nutrition, the importance of calorie reduction, the need for lifestyle adjustments and the psychological aspects of weight loss, you will equip yourself with the knowledge necessary to achieve your goals and turn over a new leaf in your life.

Join us on this journey through the basics, and take the first step on the road to a healthier, happier you.

The philosophy behind Dr. Nowzaradan's diet

At the heart of Dr. Younan Nowzaradan's approach to dieting lies a philosophy that goes far beyond the mechanical reduction of calories and targeted weight loss. It is a philosophy that emphasizes an understanding of the human body, its needs and the profound connection between our physical state and our emotional well-being. In this chapter, we dive into the foundations of this philosophy and explore how it forms the basis for a transformative journey towards health and happiness.

Holistic health as a goal

Dr. Nowzaradan does not see weight loss as an isolated goal, but as part of a broader quest for holistic health. His approach assumes that true change can only be achieved by harmonizing body and mind. He emphasizes that a healthy weight is a by-product of a balanced, nutrient-rich lifestyle that includes physical activity and emotional satisfaction.

Focus on the patient

A key aspect of Dr. Now's philosophy is the individualized approach to each patient. He recognizes that each person is unique, with individual needs, challenges and goals. This recognition of individuality is fundamental to developing a diet and lifestyle plan that is not only effective, but also sustainable.

Education as a cornerstone

Knowledge is power - a principle that Dr. Now has deeply embedded in his work. He believes that educating his patients about the basics of nutrition, how their bodies work and the psychological aspects of eating is critical to long-term success. Through education, Dr. Now empowers his patients to make informed choices and develop a sense of control over their health and well-being.

The role of personal responsibility

While Dr. Now provides his patients with advice and support, he also emphasizes the importance of personal responsibility. He believes that the path to health requires active participation - a commitment to daily choices that promote health and a willingness to overcome old habits that are detrimental to wellness.

Long-term perspective

Dr. Nowzaradan's philosophy is geared towards the long term. Quick fixes or short-term diets are not part of his approach. Instead, he emphasizes gradual, steady changes that lead to lasting improvements. He understands that true transformation takes time and that patience and perseverance are key components on the road to a healthier life.

Summary

The philosophy behind Dr. Nowzaradan's diet emphasizes the importance of a holistic view of health and weight loss. It is based on the principles of individualization, education, personal responsibility and longevity. These fundamentals not only form the basis for his patients' success, but also offer valuable insights for anyone looking to embark on the path to a healthier and more fulfilling life. By understanding and embracing this philosophy, we open the door to true change - a change that goes far beyond the number on the scale.

The scientific basis of weight loss

Understanding the science behind weight loss is essential to embarking on the path to a healthier life. This knowledge not only serves as a compass on your journey, but also as an anchor to hold you steady in moments of uncertainty or doubt. In this chapter, we highlight the scientific principles behind effective and sustainable weight loss.

Understanding energy balance

At the heart of weight loss is the concept of energy balance. The human body needs energy, which it obtains from food in the form of calories. Weight loss occurs when the body uses more energy than it takes in from food. This principle sounds simple, but its application requires a deep understanding of how different foods and activities affect this energy balance.

The role of macronutrients

Macronutrients - carbohydrates, proteins and fats - are the main sources of energy for the body. Each of these macronutrients has a specific role in the body and influences the energy balance in different ways. Proteins, for example, are essential for building and repairing body tissue and can increase feelings of satiety. Carbohydrates are the primary source of energy, while fats fulfill important functions in cell structure and hormone production. A balanced ratio of these macronutrients is crucial for healthy weight loss.

Metabolism and thermogenesis

Metabolism plays a central role in weight loss. It encompasses all chemical processes in the body that produce and consume energy. Thermogenesis, the production of heat in the body, is part of the metabolic process that burns calories. Various factors, such as genetic predisposition, diet and physical activity, can influence metabolism.

Psychological factors

Weight loss is not just a question of physiology. Psychological factors play an equally important role. Emotional eating, stress and lack of sleep can influence eating behavior and thus energy balance. Understanding these relationships helps to develop strategies that target not only the body but also the mind.

The importance of movement

Physical activity increases the body's energy consumption and is therefore an important factor in weight loss. But exercise offers more than just calorie burning; it also improves heart health, strengthens muscles and promotes mental well-being. Integrating regular exercise into everyday life is a key element for sustainable weight loss and overall health.

Summary

The science behind weight loss is complex and includes an understanding of energy balance, macronutrients, metabolism, psychological factors and the role of exercise. A sound knowledge in these areas will allow you to make informed decisions that lead to effective and lasting weight loss. By understanding the science behind weight loss, you will equip yourself with the knowledge necessary to succeed on your journey to a healthier life.

Chapter 2: The start of your journey

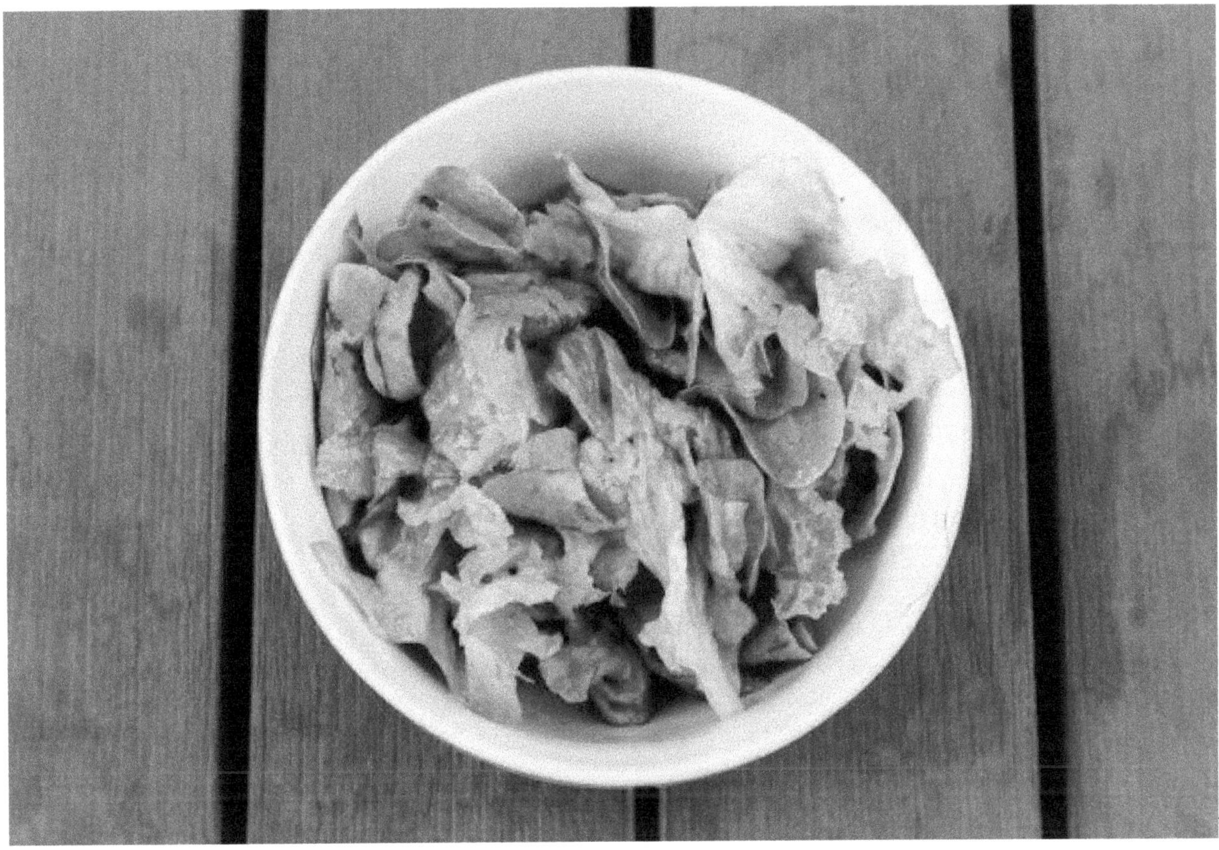

Welcome to the starting point of a journey that will not only change your physical appearance, but also your inner world. The beginning of this journey may be challenging for many, but it is also an invitation to look at your life from a new perspective and take bold steps towards health and well-being. In this chapter, we guide you through the first, crucial steps on your path to weight loss and a healthier life using Dr. Nowzaradan's method.

Preparing for success

Every big change starts with preparation. Preparing for success in your weight loss journey involves more than just deciding to lose weight. It's about creating a firm foundation on which your new habits can thrive. This means evaluating and adjusting your lifestyle, eating habits and even your environment to support your goals.

Mental strategies

The mental aspect of weight loss is just as important as the physical component. Attitude and motivation can have a significant impact on your success. In this section, we discuss how you can develop a positive attitude, mentally overcome obstacles and build strong, lasting motivation. The power of positive thinking, the importance of self-acceptance and techniques to boost your inner motivation are highlighted here.

Create a personal plan

A personalized plan tailored to your specific needs, goals and circumstances is the key to success. We will guide you through the process of goal setting, from defining realistic, achievable goals to developing a customized action plan that includes both nutrition and exercise. This plan will be your guide and companion on the road to a healthier you.

Set goals

Setting goals is an art. They need to be challenging but achievable; specific but flexible. In this section, you will learn how to define SMART (specific, measurable, achievable, relevant, time-bound) goals for your weight loss and health improvement. We'll discuss how to use short-term goals as steps towards your long-term goals and how to measure and celebrate progress.

Start the journey

With preparation, mental strategies, a personal plan and clearly defined goals, you are now ready to begin your journey. This section serves as your jumpstart - a motivating call to action. We explore how to take the first step, how to prepare for the inevitable challenges and how to stay on track in the early days and weeks.

Summary

Beginning your journey to weight loss and a healthier life is a bold step. By preparing, developing mental strategies, creating a personalized plan and setting goals, you are laying the foundation for your success. This chapter has given you the tools to move forward with confidence and clarity. Remember that every step you take is a step closer to your healthier self. Let's walk this path together.

Preparing for success: Mental strategies

Beginning a weight loss journey is not just a matter of physical adjustment, but also requires profound mental preparation. The power of our thoughts can either strengthen or hinder us on our journey. In this chapter, we focus on the mental strategies that will help set you up for success and discuss how you can create a mental foundation that will carry you through the ups and downs of your journey.

The power of a positive attitude

A positive attitude is the cornerstone of every success. It starts with believing in yourself and the conviction that change is possible. A positive attitude allows you to see challenges as opportunities for growth and setbacks as learning moments. In this section, you will learn how to recognize and transform negative self-talk and how to cultivate an optimistic outlook that motivates and inspires you.

Visualize goals

The power of visualization cannot be underestimated. By visualizing your life after successful weight loss, you create a strong mental connection to your goals. This technique anchors your goals in your subconscious and increases your motivation to achieve them. We'll show you how to use effective visualization techniques to bring your goals to life and clearly see the steps necessary to achieve them.

Self-talk and affirmations

The way we talk to ourselves has a profound impact on our self-image and our ability to achieve goals. Learn to consciously engage in positive self-talk and use affirmations to build self-confidence and overcome doubt. This section provides practical guidance on developing affirmations tailored to your specific goals and challenges.

Stress management

Stress is a common companion on the weight loss journey and can cause both physical and mental setbacks. Here we explore stress management techniques, such as deep breathing exercises, meditation and mindfulness practice, to help you maintain calm and clarity during stressful moments. The ability to manage stress effectively is crucial to staying focused and committed to your journey.

The power of community

No one is an island, and the road to weight loss is not a journey you have to take alone. Support from a community of like-minded people can make a huge difference. In this section, we discuss how you can find a supportive community and get actively involved to receive encouragement and help others. Together you can overcome challenges and celebrate shared successes.

Summary

Mental strategies are an indispensable part of your preparation for success. By cultivating a positive attitude, visualizing your goals, engaging in positive self-talk, managing stress, and harnessing the power of community, you will create a solid mental foundation for your journey. This chapter provides you with the tools to stay mentally strong, stay motivated and pursue your goals with confidence and determination. Let's start this mental journey and pave the way to a healthier life together.

Create a personal plan: Set goals

The key to successful change lies not only in the desire to improve, but also in the ability to translate that desire into concrete, actionable steps. In this chapter, we focus on how you can create a personal plan that is tailored to your individual needs, preferences and circumstances. A key aspect of this plan is goal setting - a process that provides clarity, focus and direction.

The importance of clearly defined goals

Goals give us a fixed point to work towards and help us to focus our energy and resources effectively. A clearly defined set of goals is like a map on your journey to weight loss and a healthier life. It is important that these goals are realistic and achievable to avoid discouragement and encourage a sense of progress.

Use SMART goals

The SMART principle is a proven method for setting goals. SMART stands for Specific, Measurable, Achievable, Relevant and Time-bound. By aligning your goals with these criteria, you significantly increase your chances of success. We will go through each aspect of the SMART principle and give examples of how you can apply it to your weight loss goals.

- **Specific:** Define exactly what you want to achieve. Instead of "I want to lose weight", say "I want to lose 10 kilograms in the next 6 months".
- **Measurable: Make sure** you can measure your progress. "I will track my progress by weighing myself weekly and recording my measurements."
- **Achievable:** Set yourself goals that are challenging but realistic. Take your current circumstances and resources into account.
- **Relevant:** Choose goals that are important to your personal wants and needs. "Losing weight will help me improve my health and be more active with my children."
- **Time-bound:** Set a clear deadline. "I will lose 10 kilograms by the end of the year."

Short and long-term goals

It is helpful to set both short and long-term goals. Short-term goals serve as milestones that give you motivation and a sense of accomplishment as you move toward your long-term goals. We will explore how you can create a balance between both types of goals to promote lasting change.

Develop a personalized action plan

With your SMART goals as a foundation, the next step is to create a detailed action plan. This plan should include specific strategies and tactics on how to achieve your goals, from adjusting your diet to a regular exercise program. We will discuss how you can customize your plan to overcome obstacles and respond flexibly to changes in your life.

Summary

Creating a personal plan and setting goals are crucial steps on your journey to a healthier you. By applying the SMART principle and developing a balance between short and long-term goals, you will lay a solid foundation for your success. Remind yourself that every step you take is a step closer to your goal, and that your personal plan and goals are the tools that will help you get there.

Chapter 3: The Dr. Nowzaradan Diet Plan

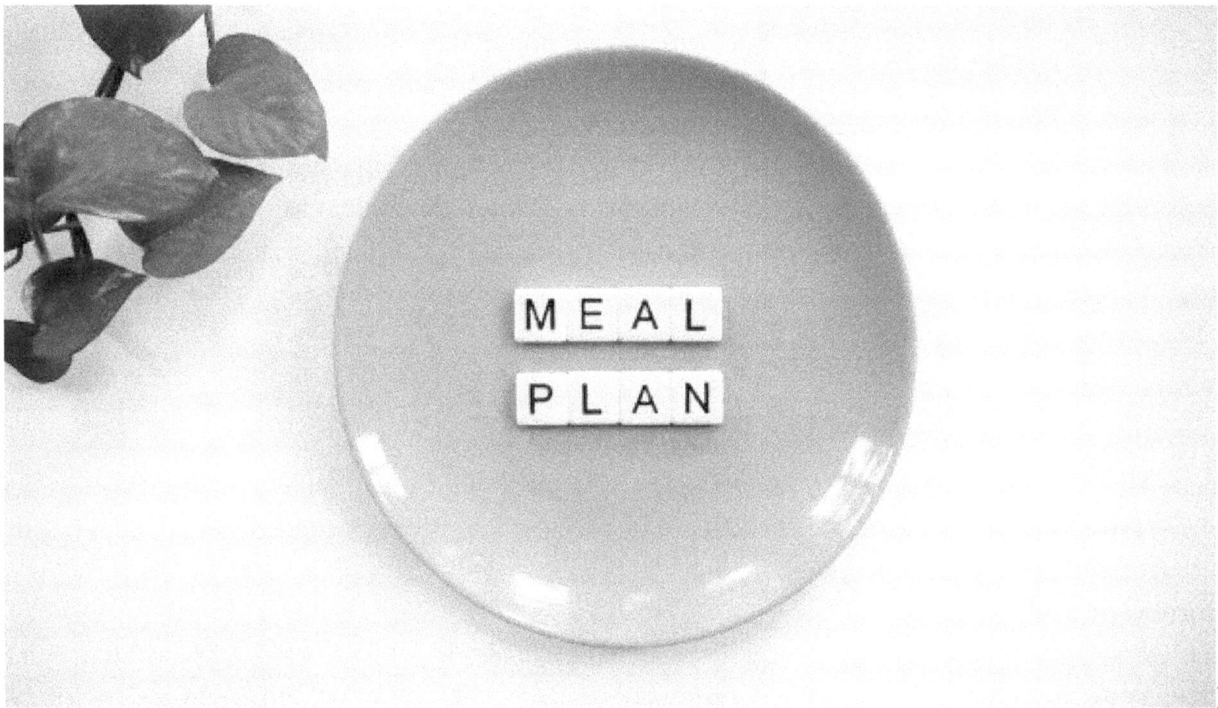

In this chapter, we reveal the core aspects of Dr. Nowzaradan's diet plan, a method that has not only helped numerous participants in the popular TV series "My 600-lb Life," but also anyone looking for a sustainable way to lose weight and improve their health. Dr. Now's approach combines strict calorie control with a deep understanding of the emotional and physical aspects of weight loss. Here we dive into the details that make this plan so effective.

Basic principles of the diet

The core of the Dr. Nowzaradan diet plan is to limit your daily calorie intake to about 1200 calories. However, this number is not set in stone; it adapts to individual needs and goals. The plan emphasizes the importance of a balanced diet that is rich in nutrients but low in empty calories and harmful fats.

What you can eat: Allowed foods

Dr. Now's diet emphasizes foods that are high in protein, low in carbohydrates and low in saturated fats. Recommended foods include:

- **Lean proteins:** Chicken, turkey, fish, egg whites and low-fat dairy products.
- **Vegetables:** A wide range of colorful vegetables, especially leafy greens and anything rich in fiber.
- **Fruits:** Fruits with a low glycemic index, which help to keep blood sugar levels stable.
- **Whole grain products:** Consumed in moderation, they provide valuable fiber and energy.
- **Healthy fats:** avocados, nuts and seeds in controlled portions.

What you should avoid: Prohibited foods

The plan recommends avoiding or severely limiting certain foods, especially those rich in simple sugars, saturated fats and excess calories. These include:

- **Sugary drinks and snacks:** soft drinks, sweets, cakes and other sugary foods.
- **High-fat foods:** fast food, fried foods and highly processed snacks.

- **White flour products:** White bread, pasta and other refined cereal products.

The importance of consistency and flexibility

While the plan provides clear guidelines, Dr. Now emphasizes the importance of flexibility. Each person is unique, and what works for one person may not necessarily be optimal for another. A willingness to adapt the plan as needed while maintaining the basic principles is critical to long-term success.

Summary

The Dr. Nowzaradan Diet Plan is more than just a simple list of dos and don'ts. It is a comprehensive approach to weight loss based on the principles of calorie control, a balanced diet and a deep understanding of each person's individual needs. By following this plan and adapting it to your personal goals and circumstances, you can start on the path to a healthier and more fulfilling life.

Basic principles of the diet

Dr. Nowzaradan's diet plan, often described as revolutionary, is actually built on simple yet powerful principles. These cornerstones serve as guidelines to help us understand our bodies, nourish them properly and build a healthy relationship with food. Below, we look at the essential principles at the core of Dr. Low's diet.

Create calorie awareness

At the forefront of Dr. Low's diet principles is calorie awareness. The idea is not to obsessively count calories, but to develop an understanding of how the quantity and quality of calories we consume affect our weight and health. Dr. Now recommends a daily calorie intake that is generally around 1200 calories, although this can be adjusted to suit individual needs. The goal is to achieve a negative energy balance, where the body burns more calories than it takes in, resulting in weight loss.

Choose nutrient-rich foods

Another key principle is the emphasis on nutrient-rich foods. Dr. Nowzaradan is adamant that his patients choose foods that provide the body with essential vitamins, minerals, proteins and other nutrients. These include lean proteins that help build muscle, complex carbohydrates for long-lasting energy and healthy fats that are important for cell function. This emphasis on nutrient density over calorie density is critical to maintaining health and wellness during weight loss.

Understanding the importance of portions

Portion control is another cornerstone of Dr. Now's diet. It is about regulating the amount of food consumed to avoid overeating and ensure adequate calorie intake. By understanding and applying portion control, patients learn to recognize and respect their feelings of fullness, which leads to healthier eating behaviors.

Plan regular meals

Creating regularity in your meals helps to boost your metabolism and maintain a stable energy level throughout the day. Dr. Now advises spreading meals throughout the day, avoiding cravings and overeating. This principle not only promotes a steady intake of nutrients, but also helps to avoid emotional eating and the calorie traps associated with it.

Taking a holistic view

Finally, Dr. Now emphasizes the importance of taking a holistic view of weight loss. He recognizes that real and lasting change requires both physical and emotional adjustments. The diet is not just a weight loss plan, but a way of life that encompasses physical activity, mental wellness and emotional resilience.

Summary

The basic principles of Dr. Nowzaradan's diet form the foundation for healthy, sustainable weight loss and improved well-being. By understanding these principles and integrating them into your everyday life, you create a solid foundation for your journey to health. It's not just about losing weight, it's about making a lasting change that will transform your life for the better.

What you can eat: Allowed foods

When approaching Dr. Nowzaradan's diet, it's easy to fall into the trap of thinking that restricting yourself to 1200 calories a day means a restrictive and monotonous diet. However, the key to success lies not in restriction, but in choice. This chapter is dedicated to the foods that are not only allowed but also recommended to nourish your body, improve your health and support you on your weight loss journey.

Lean proteins

Proteins are the building blocks of life and essential for building and maintaining muscle mass, especially important during a diet phase to boost metabolism. Dr. Now recommends lean protein sources that will help you feel fuller longer without consuming excessive calories. These include:

- Chicken breast or turkey breast without skin
- Fish, especially fatty fish such as salmon, which is rich in omega-3 fatty acids
- Eggs, with a focus on protein for those who want to pay particular attention to their fat intake
- Low-fat dairy products such as Greek yogurt or cottage cheese

Plenty of vegetables

Vegetables should form the core of your meals. They not only provide important vitamins and minerals, but also fiber, which ensures good digestion and a long-lasting feeling of satiety. Focus on a variety of colors and types:

- Green leafy vegetables such as spinach, kale and rocket
- Cruciferous vegetables such as broccoli, cauliflower and Brussels sprouts
- Colorful vegetables such as peppers, carrots and eggplants

Fruit with care

While fruits are a great source of vitamins, minerals and fiber, it's important to choose them wisely to keep an eye on your sugar balance. Fruits with a low glycemic index are ideal:

- Berries such as strawberries, blueberries and raspberries
- Apples and pears with the skin on for extra fiber
- Stone fruit such as peaches and plums in moderation

Whole grains and complex carbohydrates

Although the focus is on low carbohydrates, whole grain products and complex carbohydrates in moderate amounts are important for energy supply and satiety:

- Wholemeal bread and pasta, preferably in smaller portions
- Quinoa, bulgur and oats, which can be used in a variety of ways

Healthy fats

Fats are essential for the absorption of certain vitamins and brain health. Choose healthy fats that support your heart and brain:

- Avocado, an excellent source of monounsaturated fats
- Nuts and seeds in small quantities, such as almonds, walnuts and chia seeds
- Olive oil and other vegetable oils in moderation for cooking

Summary

The permitted foods in Dr. Nowzaradan's diet plan are selected to provide a balanced, nutrient-rich diet that supports the body while contributing to weight loss. By incorporating these foods into your daily diet, you can enjoy a diet that is not only effective, but also varied and tasty. Remember that variety and moderation are the keys to successful and sustainable weight loss.

What you should avoid: Prohibited foods

While the Dr. Nowzaradan diet plan highlights a variety of nutritious and healthy foods, there are also certain foods that are on the "forbidden" list. These foods are usually high in empty calories, saturated fats or simple sugars, which can hinder the weight loss process. In this chapter, we highlight which foods you should avoid and why.

Sugary drinks and snacks

Sugary drinks such as soft drinks, fruit juices and energy drinks are often loaded with simple sugars that quickly enter the bloodstream and spike insulin levels. This can not only lead to weight gain, but also increases the risk of type 2 diabetes and other metabolic diseases. The situation is similar with high-sugar snacks such as sweets, cookies and cakes, which often offer little nutritional value besides sugar.

High-fat foods

High-fat foods, especially those high in saturated fats such as fast food, fried snacks and processed meat products, should be avoided. Saturated fats can raise cholesterol levels and increase the risk of heart disease. They are also calorie dense and can make it difficult to achieve a negative energy balance.

White flour products

Products made from white flour, such as white bread, pasta and pastries, are low in fiber and nutrients. They can quickly raise blood sugar levels and lead to a subsequent drop, which can promote cravings. Eating whole grain products is a better alternative, as they keep you full for longer and make a positive contribution to your health.

Highly processed foods

Highly processed foods are often high in sugar, salt and artificial additives, while being low in essential nutrients. These products include potato chips, crackers and ready meals. They can hinder weight loss and often have a negative impact on overall health.

Certain fats and oils

While healthy fats are an important part of the diet, certain fats and oils, especially trans fats and some saturated fats, should be avoided. Trans fats are found in some margarines, baked goods and many convenience foods and can increase the risk of heart disease.

Summary

Avoiding certain foods is an essential part of Dr. Nowzaradan's diet plan. By eliminating sugary drinks and snacks, high-fat foods, white flour products, highly processed foods, and certain fats and oils from your diet, you can not only reach your weight loss goal more effectively, but also improve your overall health. It's about making conscious choices that nourish and support your body, rather than loading it with empty calories and harmful substances.

30-day diet plan

To give you a practical guide to what Dr. Nowzaradan's diet might look like, we have created a 30-day diet plan consisting of 3 main meals and a snack.

This eating plan is designed to illustrate the principles of a balanced, nutrient-dense, low-calorie diet that supports the body and promotes weight control.

Dr. Nowzaradan's diet plan is based on a calorie intake of 1,200 Kcal per day. However, this does not mean that you have to consume a maximum of 1,200 kcal. The number of kcal you need to consume varies from person to person. You will therefore need to adjust the portions in the recipes accordingly.

Nevertheless, there are some basic rules that you should always keep in mind.

Adjust portion sizes: Depending on individual calorie requirements and activity levels, portion sizes should be adjusted to control total calorie intake.

Drink water: Make sure you drink enough water every day to stay hydrated.

Day 1:

- **Breakfast:** Avocado toast on wholemeal bread *(Pg. 62)*
- **Lunch:** Eggplant lasagna with ricotta and spinach *(Pg. 76)*
- **Dinner:** Pike-perch fillet on a bed of lentils *(Pg. 113)*

Day 2:

- **Brcakfast:** Chia pudding with coconut *(Pg. 62)*
- **Lunch:** Cauliflower rice with chicken and vegetables *(Pg. 76)*
- **Dinner:** Spicy pumpkin stew with chicken *(Pg. 112)*

Day 3:

- **Breakfast:** Protein wraps with lean turkey bacon *(Pg. 63)*
- **Lunch:** Broccoli quiche without base *(Pg. 77)*
- **Dinner:** Zucchini noodles with avocado pesto *(Pg. 114)*

Day 4:

- **Breakfast:** Muesli with low-fat milk and fresh fruit *(Pg. 70)*
- **Lunch:** Cod fillet with broccoli and almonds *(Pg. 84)*
- **Dinner:** Baked cauliflower with parmesan *(Pg. 111)*

Day 5:

- **Breakfast:** Boiled eggs and asparagus salad *(Pg. 64)*
- **Lunch:** Vegetarian zucchini lasagna *(Pg. 112)*
- **Dinner:** Lamb's lettuce with grilled salmon *(Pg. 99)*

Day 6:

- **Breakfast:** Protein smoothie with spinach and berries *(Pg. 72)*
- **Lunch:** Vegetable pan with prawns *(Pg. 82)*
- **Dinner:** Chicken breast with ratatouille *(Pg. 101)*

Day 7:

- **Breakfast:** Oatmeal with apple and cinnamon *(Pg. 67)*
- **Lunch:** Cucumber and tomato salad with cottage cheese *(Pg. 83)*
- **Dinner:** Roast chicken with broccoli and almonds *(Pg. 80)*

Day 8:

- **Breakfast:** Quinoa breakfast bowl with berries *(Pg. 72)*
- **Lunch:** Chicken breast on rocket with balsamic dressing *(Pg. 84)*
- **Dinner:** Mediterranean vegetable casserole *(Pg. 105)*

Day 9:

- **Breakfast:** Lentil and spinach breakfast pans *(Pg. 68)*
- **Lunch:** Colorful lentil salad with feta and fresh herbs *(Pg. 78)*
- **Dinner:** Tuna steak with Mediterranean vegetables *(Pg. 110)*

Day 10:

- **Breakfast:** Omelette with spinach and feta *(Pg. 70)*
- **Lunch:** Mushroom and spinach omelette *(Pg. 16)*
- **Dinner:** Zucchini spaghetti with turkey bolognese *(Pg. 16)*

Day 11:

- **Breakfast:** Pumpkin and oatmeal porridge *(Pg. 67)*
- **Lunch:** Tuna salad with avocado and egg *(Pg. 79)*
- **Dinner:** Spicy pumpkin stew with chicken *(Pg. 112)*

Day 12:

- **Breakfast:** Pancakes made with wholemeal buttermilk *(Pg. 71)*
- **Lunch:** Vegetable broth with chicken strips *(Pg. 81)*
- **Dinner:** Vegetarian zucchini lasagna *(Pg. 112)*

Day 13:

- **Breakfast:** Zucchini muffins (sugar-free) *(Pg. 75)*

- **Lunch:** Chicken breast on rocket with balsamic dressing *(Pg. 84)*
- **Dinner:** Eggplant rolls with ricotta and spinach *(Pg. 96)*

Day 14:

- **Breakfast:** Roasted chickpeas and avocado salad *(Pg. 65)*
- **Lunch:** Chickpea salad with peppers and onions *(Pg. 86)*
- **Dinner:** Cod fillet in a bed of vegetables *(Pg. 98)*

Day 15:

- **Breakfast:** Salmon fillet with asparagus and lemon butter *(Pg. 87)*
- **Lunch:** Spinach and feta pancakes (without flour) *(Pg. 16)*
- **Dinner:** Roast chicken with broccoli and almonds *(Pg. 16)*

Day 16:

- **Breakfast:** Chia pudding with coconut *(Pg. 62)*
- **Lunch:** Cauliflower steak with chimichurri sauce *(Pg. 91)*
- **Dinner:** Zucchini noodles with avocado pesto *(Pg. 114)*

Day 17:

- **Breakfast:** Avocado toast on wholemeal bread *(Pg. 62)*
- **Lunch:** Vegetable pan with prawns *(Pg. 82)*
- **Dinner:** Spicy pumpkin stew with chicken *(Pg. 112)*

Day 18:

- **Breakfast:** Muesli with low-fat milk and fresh fruit *(Pg. 70)*
- **Lunch:** Cucumber and tomato salad with cottage cheese *(Pg. 83)*
- **Dinner:** Baked cauliflower with parmesan *(Pg. 111)*

Day 19:

- **Breakfast:** Tofu scramble with vegetables *(Pg. 74)*
- **Lunch:** Mediterranean vegetable casserole *(Pg. 16)*
- **Dinner:** Low-calorie turkey goulash with peppers *(Pg. 16)*

Day 20:

- **Breakfast:** Protein smoothie with spinach and berries *(Pg. 72)*

- **Lunch:** Mediterranean vegetable casserole *(Pg. 87)*
- **Dinner:** Salmon fillet with green asparagus and quinoa *(Pg. 104)*

Day 21:

- **Breakfast:** Boiled eggs and asparagus salad *(Pg. 64)*
- **Lunch:** Mushroom and spinach omelette *(Pg. 79)*
- **Dinner:** Tuna steak with Mediterranean vegetables *(Pg. 92)*

Day 22:

- **Breakfast:** Oatmeal with apple and cinnamon *(Pg. 67)*
- **Lunch:** Cucumber and tomato salad with cottage cheese *(Pg. 83)*
- **Dinner:** Roast chicken with broccoli and almonds *(Pg. 80)*

Day 23:

- **Breakfast:** Lentil and spinach breakfast pancakes *(Pg. 68)*
- **Lunch:** Cod fillet with broccoli and almonds *(Pg. 84)*
- **Dinner:** Vegetarian zucchini lasagna *(Pg. 112)*

Day 24:

- **Breakfast:** Muesli with low-fat milk and fresh fruit *(Pg. 70)*
- **Lunch:** Vegetable pan with prawns *(Pg. 82)*
- **Dinner:** Spicy pumpkin stew with chicken *(Pg. 112)*

Day 25:

- **Breakfast:** Zucchini muffins (sugar-free) *(Pg. 75)*
- **Lunch:** Cauliflower rice with chicken and vegetables *(Pg. 76)*
- **Dinner:** Baked cauliflower with parmesan *(Pg. 111)*

Day 26:

- **Breakfast:** Chia pudding with coconut *(Pg. 62)*
- **Lunch:** Chicken breast on rocket with balsamic dressing *(Pg. 84)*
- **Dinner:** Zucchini noodles with avocado pesto *(Pg. 114)*

Day 27:

- **Breakfast:** Avocado toast on wholemeal bread *(Pg. 62)*
- **Lunch:** Vegetarian zucchini lasagna *(Pg. 112)*

- **Dinner:** Lamb's lettuce with grilled salmon *(Pg. 99)*

Day 28:

- **Breakfast:** Pancakes made with wholemeal buttermilk *(Pg. 71)*
- **Lunch:** Broccoli quiche without base *(Pg. 77)*
- **Dinner:** Boiled eggs and asparagus salad *(Pg. 64)*

Day 29:

- **Breakfast:** Protein smoothie with spinach and berries *(Pg. 72)*
- **Lunch:** Colorful lentil salad with feta and fresh herbs *(Pg. 78)*
- **Dinner:** Eggplant rolls with ricotta and spinach *(Pg. 96)*

Day 30:

- **Breakfast:** Quinoa breakfast bowl with berries *(Pg. 72)*
- **Lunch:** Cucumber and tomato salad with cottage cheese *(Pg. 83)*
- **Dinner:** Pike-perch fillet on a bed of lentils *(Pg. 113)*

Shopping lists and meal preparation tips

Careful planning and preparation of your meals can make all the difference when it comes to establishing and maintaining healthy eating habits. With a well thought out shopping list and some handy meal prep tips, you'll not only save time and money, but also ensure you reach your nutritional goals. Here you will find instructions to make your week stress-free and healthy.

Create a shopping list

1. plan your meals in advance: Take time each week to plan your meals. Include breakfast, lunch, dinner and snacks.

2. list the ingredients: write down all the ingredients you need for your planned meals. Don't forget to check staples such as spices, oils and stock to see what needs to be replenished.

3. organize the list by category: Divide your list into categories such as vegetables, fruits, proteins, dairy products and dry goods. This will make shopping easier and prevent you from forgetting anything.

4 Consider seasonal produce: Incorporate seasonal foods into your meal planning to take advantage of fresher ingredients and often lower prices.

Meal preparation tips

1. choose a preparation day: choose a day of the week (e.g. Sunday) when you have time to prepare and cook meals. This can help you save time during the week.

2. use versatile ingredients: Choose ingredients that can be used in multiple recipes. For example, roasted vegetables can be used as a side dish, in salads or as a filling for wraps.

3. cook in large quantities: Prepare larger quantities of your favorite dishes and freeze portions or store them in the fridge. This way you will always have a healthy meal to hand.

4. prepare snacks: pack healthy snacks such as sliced vegetables, nuts or yogurt in advance so that you can access them quickly when you are hungry.

5. use reusable containers: Invest in high-quality, reusable containers to keep your meals and snacks fresh. This also makes it easier to take meals to work or school.

6. stay flexible: Although planning is important, stay flexible and adjust your meals if plans change or you feel like doing something else.

Summary

The keys to meal prep success are planning, organization and flexibility. A well thought out shopping list will help you shop efficiently and ensure you have all the necessary ingredients for your planned meals. By allowing time for preparation and preparing meals in advance, you can encourage healthy eating habits and increase the likelihood of eating well even during stressful times.

Chapter 4: Adjustments for your lifestyle

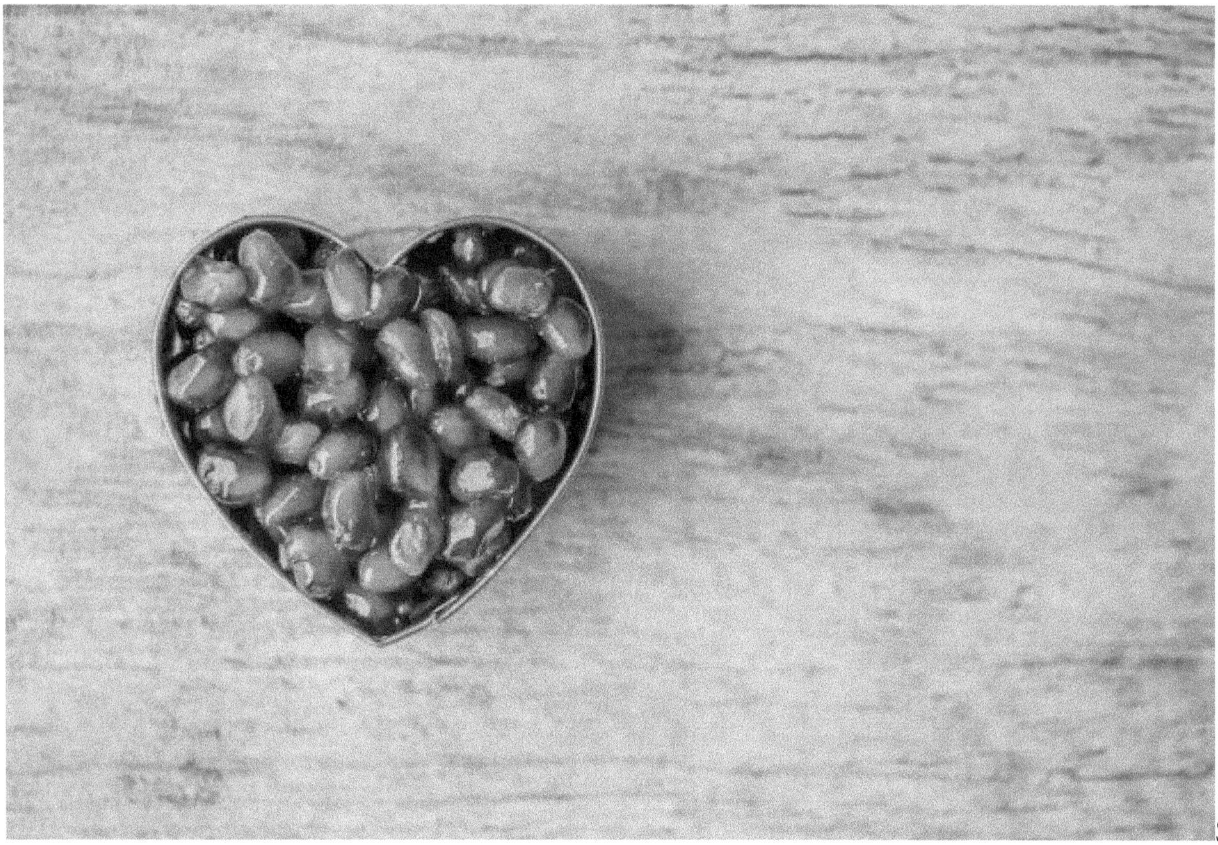

Successful weight loss and achieving a healthier lifestyle depends not only on the right diet, but also on how well that diet can be integrated into your everyday life. Everyone leads a unique life, characterized by individual routines, commitments and preferences. In this chapter, we'll show you how to adapt the Dr. Nowzaradan diet plan to different lifestyles to ensure that your efforts to eat healthier are sustainable and workable.

For employees: time management tips

In today's fast-paced world, finding time to prepare healthy meals can be a challenge. Here are some strategies that can help you:

- **Meal Prep:** Dedicate part of the weekend to preparing meals for the week ahead. Cook in large quantities and portion the meals into convenient containers.
- **Simple recipes:** Choose recipes with few ingredients that are quick and easy to prepare.
- **Use of kitchen gadgets:** Slow stoves, Instant Pots and Air Fryers can save time and make it easier to prepare healthy meals.

For families: healthy meals for everyone

Ensuring a healthy diet for the whole family can be a challenge, especially when children are involved. Here are some tips to get everyone in the family involved:

- **Plan meals together: Involve** all family members in the planning to ensure that everyone has something to eat that they like.
- **Cooking evenings:** Make cooking a family activity to spark interest in healthy foods.

- **Healthy snacks:** Keep healthy snack options to hand to resist the temptation of unhealthy alternatives.

For individuals: Simple and quick recipes

Do you live alone? No problem! Following a healthy diet can also be easy and tasty for individuals:

- **Portion control:** Invest in smaller plates and bowls to control portion sizes.
- **Social cooking:** Invite friends over to cook together to keep the social element of the meal.
- **Variety is the key:** experiment with different recipes to make meals exciting and varied.

Adaptations for special nutritional requirements

Whether for medical reasons, allergies or personal preferences - sometimes special dietary adjustments are necessary:

- **Gluten-free, lactose-free, vegetarian/vegan: There are** numerous recipes and substitutes that meet these needs while following the guidelines of the Dr. Nowzaradan diet plan.
- **Consultation with a nutritionist:** For more complex nutritional needs, professional advice can help to adapt the diet plan accordingly.

Summary

The key to successful and sustainable weight loss lies in adapting your diet plan to your individual lifestyle. Whether you are a busy professional, part of a family or someone who has special dietary needs, there are always ways to incorporate healthy eating habits into your daily routine. By applying the tips and strategies above, you can ensure that your efforts towards better health and weight loss are successful in the long run .

For employees: Time management tips

In a world where the clock always seems to be ticking against us, sticking to a healthy diet like Dr. Nowzaradan's can be a real challenge. Especially for working professionals juggling work, family and personal commitments, preparing nutritious meals may seem like a distant dream. But with the right time management strategies, you can make room for healthy eating even in a busy schedule. Here are some tips on how you can achieve this.

Set priorities

Start by recognizing that your health is a priority. This may sound obvious, but it's crucial to realize that making time to prepare healthy meals is just as important as any meeting or other commitment on your calendar. Set fixed times for meal prep, just as you would for other important tasks.

Meal Prep: A game changer

Meal prep, preparing and cooking meals in advance, is an effective way to ensure you have healthy options on hand throughout the week. Choose one day of the week - Sunday, for example - to prepare meals for the days ahead. Cook in bulk and portion the meals into individual containers. This way you always have a quick and healthy option to hand, even when time is short.

Quick and easy recipes

Not every meal has to be a culinary masterpiece. Gather a selection of simple recipes that are quick to prepare yet nutritious and tasty. Dishes that are ready in less than 30 minutes can be a lifesaver on particularly hectic days. Think salads, stews or simple stir-fries that use minimal ingredients.

Using kitchen gadgets

Modern kitchen appliances can make preparing healthy meals much easier. A slow stove, Instant Pot or Air Fryer can help you save time while still enjoying nutritious meals. Many of these appliances offer the option of adding ingredients in the morning and coming home to a ready meal in the evening.

Choose snacks wisely

For those days when even reheating a prepared meal seems too time-consuming, it's important to have healthy snacks to hand. Instead of reaching for potato chips or chocolate, choose snacks that will fill you up and give you energy without blowing your calorie balance. Think nuts, yogurt, fresh fruit or vegetable sticks with hummus.

Summary

For busy people, sticking to a healthy diet can be a challenge, but with the right time management strategies, it's entirely doable. By prioritizing your health, effective meal prep, choosing simple recipes, using modern kitchen appliances and choosing snacks wisely, you can ensure that you eat well even on hectic days. Remember that any investment in your health is an investment in your future.

Chapter 5: Overcoming challenges

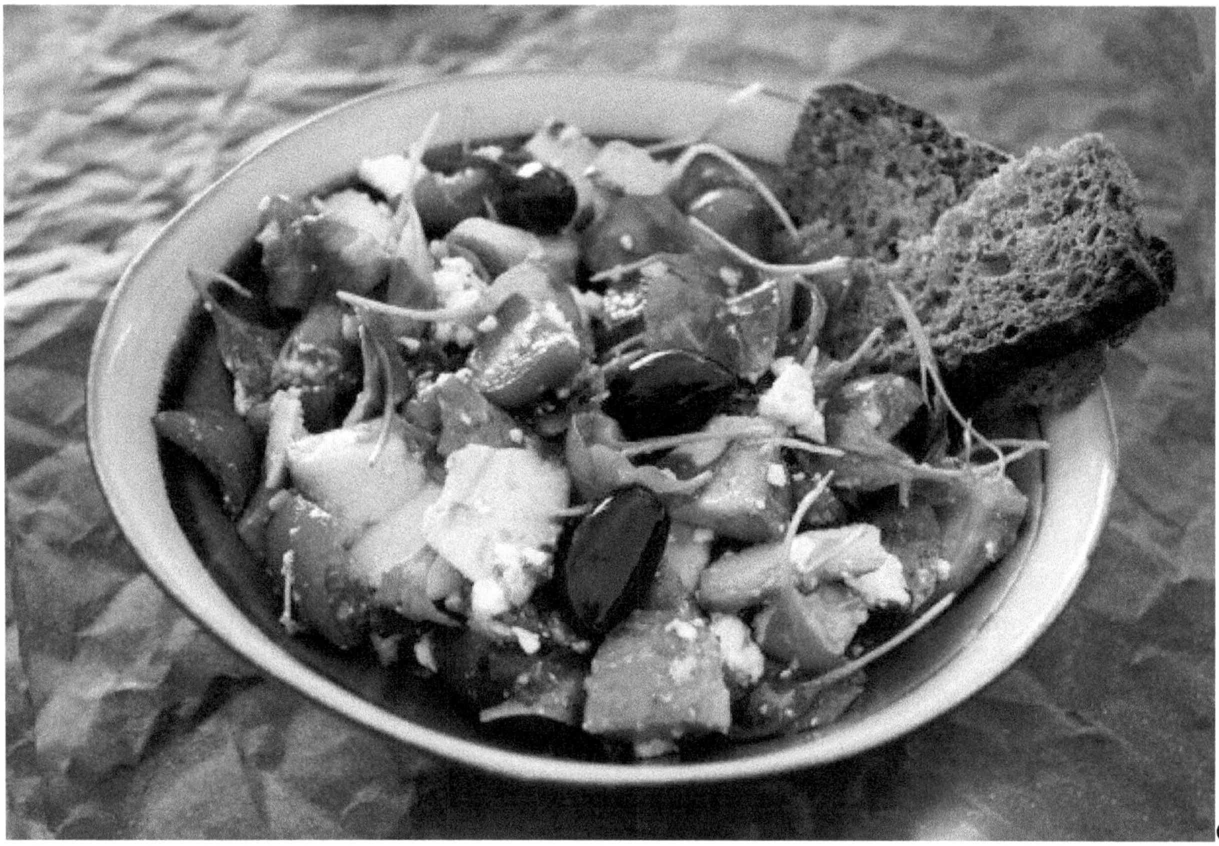

Challenges are inevitable on the path to a healthier you. They are not only part of the process, but also opportunities for growth and self-discovery. Throughout your journey with Dr. Nowzaradan's diet plan, you will encounter various obstacles, both physical and mental. In this chapter, we address the most common challenges and offer practical solutions and strategies to effectively overcome them.

Mastering cravings

Cravings can be a major obstacle on the road to weight loss. It is often not a signal from the body for real hunger, but a reaction to emotional needs, stress or boredom.

Strategies for coping:

- Identify triggers for your cravings and develop alternative coping strategies, such as going for a walk, deep breathing exercises or a hobby.
- Keep healthy snacks to hand so you don't give in to the temptation of unhealthy options.
- Drink a glass of water, as thirst is often misinterpreted as hunger.

Navigating social events

Social events can be particularly challenging as they often involve food that doesn't fit into your diet plan.

Strategies for coping:

- Eat a small, healthy meal before you go to an event to avoid feeling hungry.
- Offer to bring a healthy dish for you and others to enjoy.
- Focus on the social aspects of the event, not the food.

Maintain motivation
There may be days when your motivation wanes and achieving your goals seems unattainable.
Strategies for coping:

- Set yourself smaller, achievable goals and celebrate every success.
- Seek support from friends, family or a self-help group.
- Remind yourself of your reasons for starting this journey and visualize your successes.

Dealing with plateaus
Weight loss plateaus are normal, but can be frustrating if the scales don't budge despite your best efforts.
Strategies for coping:

- Check and adjust your diet and exercise plan.
- Increase the intensity or variability of your physical activity.
- Be patient and consistent. Plateaus are often temporary.

Coping with emotional eating
Eating in response to emotions rather than hunger can significantly impair progress.
Strategies for coping:

- Keep a food diary to identify emotional eating.
- Develop non-eating-related strategies for coping with stress and emotions, such as meditation or journaling.
- Seek professional help if you find that emotional eating is affecting your quality of life.

Summary

Challenges on your path are not only unavoidable, they are also an integral part of the learning and growth process. By facing these challenges and developing strategies to overcome them, you build resilience and move step by step towards your goals. Remind yourself that every day is a new opportunity to continue on your path, regardless of the obstacles you may have already experienced.

Common obstacles and how to overcome them

On the journey to a healthier lifestyle, you will inevitably encounter obstacles that can challenge your determination and progress. However, these challenges are not insurmountable. By understanding what these obstacles are and how to effectively address them, we strengthen our ability to stay on the path to health and wellness. Here we discuss some of the most common obstacles and offer strategies for overcoming them.

1. **Lack of time**

The obstacle: In a hectic everyday life, it can be difficult to find time to prepare healthy meals or exercise regularly.

The conquest: Plan your week in advance. Use meal prepping to prepare healthy meals and incorporate short but effective workouts into your daily routine. Even 10 minutes of intense exercise can make a difference.

1. **Lack of motivation**

The obstacle: there are days when motivation wanes and the couch seems more tempting than the gym.

The overcoming: Set clear, achievable goals and remind yourself regularly of your reasons for starting. Find an accountability partner or join a support group to stay motivated.

1. **Social pressure**

The obstacle: Social occasions and pressure from family or friends can make it difficult to make healthy choices.

Overcoming: Communicate openly about your goals and seek support from your social circle. Offer to contribute healthy alternatives to social gatherings or suggest activity-based gatherings instead of food-centered gatherings.

1. **Emotional eating**

The obstacle: Stress, boredom or emotional turmoil often lead to emotional eating, which can undermine your goals.

Overcoming: Develop an awareness of your emotional eating habits. Look for other ways to deal with your feelings, such as through exercise, hobbies or talking to friends.

1. **Unrealistic expectations**

The obstacle: Setting unrealistic goals or expecting immediate results can lead to frustration and discouragement.

Overcoming: Be patient with yourself and set realistic, measurable goals. Understand that progress takes time and that every small change counts.

1. **Weight loss plateaus**

The obstacle: Despite initial success, it can happen that the weight suddenly stagnates, which can have a demotivating effect.

The overcoming: Recognize that plateaus are a normal part of the weight loss process. Review your diet and exercise and adjust as needed. Sometimes patience is simply required.

1. **Information overload**

The obstacle: The abundance of diet information and advice can be overwhelming and lead to confusion.

Overcoming it: Concentrate on proven principles of healthy eating and exercise and avoid fad diets or quick fixes. Seek professional advice if necessary.

For families: healthy meals for everyone

Integrating healthy meals into everyday family life can be a challenge, especially when each family member has different tastes and preferences. Switching to a diet that follows Dr. Nowzaradan's principles requires not only creativity and planning, but also the commitment of all family members. In this chapter, you will learn how to prepare healthy meals for the whole family that are not only nutritious but also delicious.

Laying the foundation

It starts with the understanding that healthy eating is an investment in the future of every family member. The basis for successful implementation is the involvement of everyone in the planning and preparation of meals. This not only promotes interest in healthy eating, but also strengthens family cohesion.

Joint planning and preparation

A weekly planning meeting to discuss menus and assign tasks can work wonders. Let children help choose the recipes and involve them in the preparation. This not only teaches them important cooking skills, but also helps them develop an appreciation for the ingredients and the process of food preparation.

Education is the key

Use mealtimes as an opportunity to talk about the benefits of a healthy diet. Explain how certain foods strengthen the body and why it is important to avoid certain others. Simple explanations and setting examples can have a profound impact on your children's eating habits.

Adaptation to individual needs

Recognize individual needs and preferences and try to incorporate these into meals. This may mean offering variations on some dishes. For example, a basic dish such as baked chicken can be easily adapted for those who don't like skin by removing the skin before serving.

Healthy snacks and alternatives

A selection of healthy snacks that are easily accessible can reduce the need for less healthy options. Fresh fruit, veggie sticks with hummus or yogurt are great snacks that provide energy without leading to excess calories. Experiment with healthy alternatives to family favorites, like whole wheat pizza with veggies or homemade butterless popcorn.

Flexibility and patience

Not every meal will be a hit right away, and that's okay. Flexibility and patience are key as you acclimate your family to a healthier lifestyle. Celebrate the small victories, like when a picky eater tries a new vegetable, and be ready to make adjustments as needed.

Summary

Creating healthy meals for the whole family requires commitment, creativity and a willingness to experiment and learn. By making meal planning and preparation a community activity, you are building a solid foundation for healthy eating habits that can last a lifetime. Remember that transitioning to a healthier lifestyle is a journey that requires patience, but the rewards - a healthier, happier family life - are priceless.

Chapter 6: Fitness and exercise

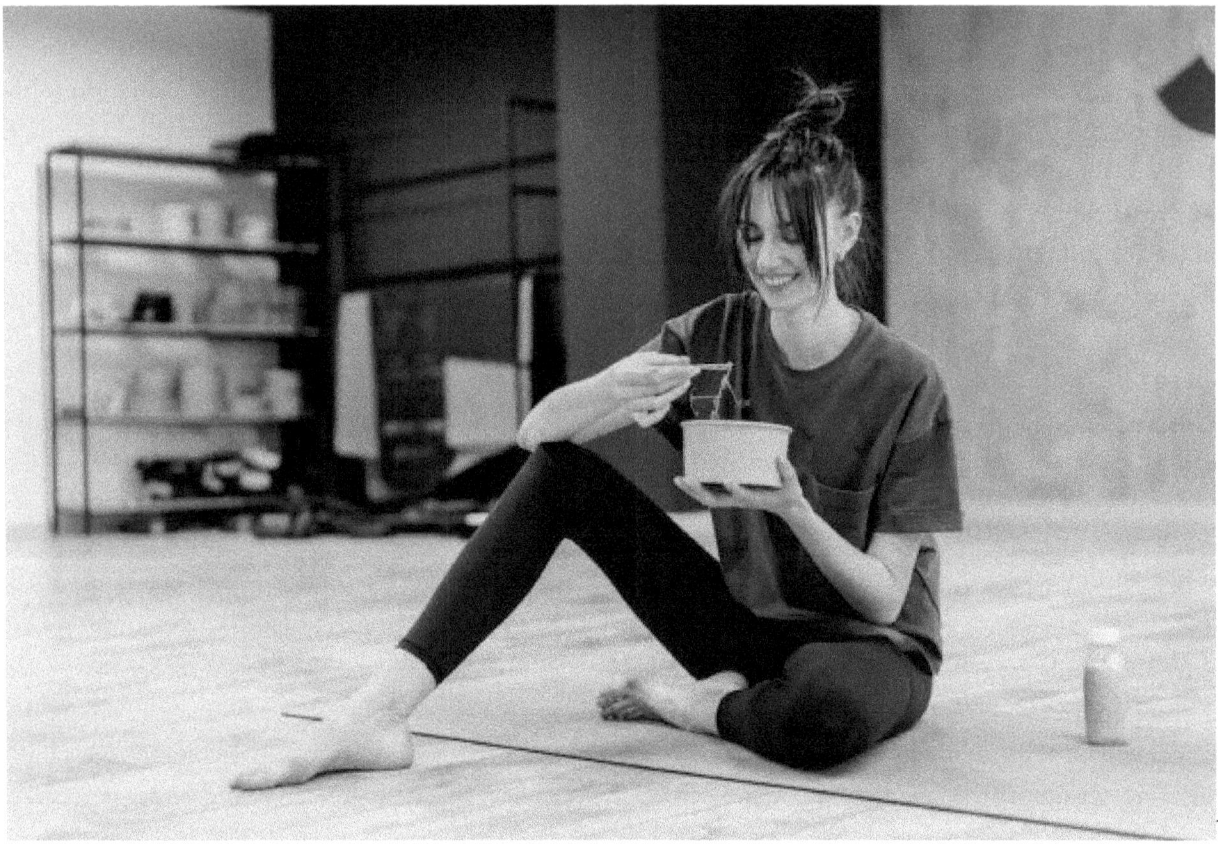

While a balanced diet lays the foundation for weight loss and overall wellness, regular physical activity completes the puzzle of a healthy lifestyle. Fitness and exercise are essential to not only burn calories, but also strengthen the body, improve mood and reduce the risk of chronic disease. In this chapter, we explore how you can incorporate exercise into your daily routine to get the most out of the benefits of the Dr. Nowzaradan Diet Plan.

The importance of regular exercise

Regular physical activity has multiple health benefits that go beyond simply burning calories. It improves heart health, strengthens bones and muscles, promotes mental health and can even improve sleep quality. In addition, exercise can help accelerate weight loss and, more importantly, keep the lost weight off long term.

Adaptation to your fitness level

It is important to choose an exercise program that suits your current fitness level. For beginners, this may mean starting with short walks and gradually increasing the duration and intensity. People who are already active could add interval training or strength training to their program. Listen to your body and avoid overexertion to prevent injury.

Diversity is the key

To avoid boredom and challenge the whole body, it is important to add variety to your exercise program. Combine aerobic exercises such as running, swimming or cycling with strength training to build muscle and boost your metabolism. Don't forget to include flexibility and balance exercises such as yoga or Pilates, which contribute to overall fitness and reduce the risk of injury.

Integrating exercise into everyday life

Fitness doesn't always have to take place in the gym. There are many ways to integrate exercise into your everyday life. Take the stairs instead of the elevator, go for a walk during your lunch break or cycle to work if possible. Even short bursts of activity throughout the day can have a positive effect on your health.

The role of motivation

Finding the motivation to stay active on a regular basis can be a challenge. Set realistic goals, find an activity you enjoy, and look for a workout buddy to keep motivation high. Reward yourself for milestones achieved, but avoid rewards that work against your health, such as unhealthy foods.

Summary

Fitness and exercise are essential components of a healthy lifestyle and complement the nutritional guidelines of the Dr. Nowzaradan Diet Plan. By making regular physical activity a regular part of your life, you can not only lose and maintain weight, but also improve your overall health and well-being. Remember that the key to success is consistency - find activities you enjoy and make exercise a habit you love to maintain.

The importance of exercise in the diet

Incorporating regular physical activity into your diet plan isn't just a recommendation - it's a necessity for lasting success and overall wellness. While diet is the biggest part of weight loss, exercise plays a crucial role in shaping the body, improving health and increasing mental balance. In this chapter, we look at why exercise is an essential part of Dr. Nowzaradan's diet plan and how it can help you achieve your goals.

Exercise as a catalyst for weight loss

Exercise increases calorie expenditure, which can accelerate weight loss by creating a greater calorie deficit. In addition, regular exercise helps to boost your metabolism, which means that your body burns calories more efficiently even when you are at rest. But the benefits of exercise go far beyond simply burning calories.

Muscle building and body toning

During the diet, it is important not only to lose fat, but also to maintain and build muscle mass. Muscles are metabolically active, which means that they burn calories even when at rest. Strength training or resistance exercises are crucial to promote muscle building and counteract the loss of muscle mass that often accompanies calorie restriction.

Improving mental health

Regular physical activity has been proven to have positive effects on mental health. Exercise releases endorphins, the so-called 'happy hormones', which can reduce stress and improve overall wellbeing. This mental boost is especially valuable while dieting, when you may be facing challenges or moments of discouragement.

Increase in energy and well-being

Many people report a significant increase in energy and vitality when they exercise regularly. This increased energy can help you to be more active and feel more motivated to stick to your diet plan. In addition, physical activity improves sleep quality, which is crucial for recovery and regeneration of the body.

Integration into everyday life

Exercise doesn't have to mean spending hours in the gym. It's about finding ways to be more active in your daily life - be it through walking, cycling instead of driving, climbing stairs or taking short active breaks during the working day. The goal is to make exercise a natural and enjoyable part of your life.

Summary

The role of exercise in Dr. Nowzaradan's diet is undeniable. Not only does it promote more effective weight loss and body toning, but it also contributes significantly to mental strength and overall well-being. By making exercise an integral part of your diet plan, you are building a solid foundation for long-term health and happiness. Remember that every step counts - choose activities you enjoy and make exercise a constant companion on your journey to a healthier you.

Simple exercises for beginners

Getting into a regular exercise program can seem overwhelming for beginners, especially if you feel unsure of where or how to start. But the good news is that the foundation for an effective fitness routine can be laid with some simple exercises that require no special equipment and can be done anywhere. In this chapter, we'll introduce you to simple exercises designed specifically for beginners to help you get started on your fitness journey.

1. going for a walk

One of the easiest and most effective ways to start regular exercise is walking. It's easy on the joints, requires no equipment and can be adapted to your fitness level. Start with short walks of 10-15 minutes and gradually increase the duration and pace to improve your stamina.

2. squats

Squats are an excellent exercise to strengthen your legs and buttocks. Stand with your feet shoulder-width apart, stretch your arms out in front of you and bend your knees as if you were sitting on a chair. Make sure that your knees do not extend beyond the tips of your toes. The aim is to go deeper into the squat over time and increase the repetitions.

3. push-ups against the wall

Traditional push-ups can be a challenge for beginners. An alternative is to do push-ups against the wall, which strengthens the upper body, shoulders and arms without overstraining them. Stand in front of a wall at a suitable distance, place your hands at shoulder height against the wall and perform a movement similar to a push-up.

4. planks

Planks are an effective exercise to strengthen the core. Start in the push-up position and keep your body in a straight line while tensing your abdominal muscles. Hold this position for 15-30 seconds at first and gradually increase the duration to improve your core strength.

5. leg lift

Leg raises strengthen the lower abdominal muscles and are a simple exercise that is performed lying on your back. Slowly lift your straight legs off the floor and lower them again without putting them down completely. Start with a few repetitions and gradually increase the number.

6. stretching

Stretching exercises are an important part of any fitness routine to improve flexibility and reduce the risk of injury. Incorporate simple stretching exercises for all major muscle groups into your routine to improve your flexibility and relieve muscle tension.

Summary

These simple exercises are the perfect starting point for beginners to immerse themselves in the world of fitness. By regularly incorporating these exercises into your daily routine, you can build a solid foundation of physical activity and take positive steps towards your health and fitness goals. Remember to listen to your body and adjust your workouts accordingly to avoid overexertion. With patience and consistency, you will see progress and be on your way to a more active and healthy lifestyle.

How to stay fit without an expensive gym

The idea that an effective fitness routine necessarily requires a gym or expensive equipment discourages many people from even starting to exercise. But the truth is, you don't have to dig deep into your pockets to get fit. There are numerous ways you can stay fit without an expensive gym. In this chapter, we explore simple and inexpensive ways to achieve your fitness goals and maintain a healthy lifestyle.

Use your own body weight

Exercises that use only your own body weight can be incredibly effective for improving strength, endurance and flexibility. Classic examples such as squats, push-ups, planks or burpees require no equipment and can be done anywhere. Put together a routine that targets different muscle groups and you have a comprehensive workout at no cost.

Discover nature

Nature offers a fantastic and free backdrop for your training. Whether it's running, hiking, cycling or swimming, there are many ways to exercise outdoors, with the added benefit of enjoying fresh air and getting in touch with nature. Find trails or parks near you and turn the world into your gym.

Online workout resources

The internet is a goldmine of free workout guides, videos and plans. From yoga and Pilates to high-intensity interval training (HIIT), there are online offerings for every interest and fitness level. Many trainers and fitness communities offer free sessions on platforms such as YouTube, which are a great resource to use at home.

Turn everyday activities into exercise

You don't always have to schedule a special time for workouts. Integrate exercise into your everyday life, for example by walking or cycling more often instead of taking the car. Take the stairs instead of the elevator and go for walks during your lunch break. These small changes can add up to significant fitness improvements over time.

Start a training group

Exercising together with friends or family can not only be more motivating, but also fun and free. Organize regular get-togethers for joint workouts, running groups or yoga sessions in the park. The mutual motivation and support can make a big difference to your fitness routine.

Be creative with household remedies

Many everyday objects can be used as substitutes for fitness equipment. Water bottles as weights, a sturdy chair for tricep dips or a towel as a resistance band - be creative and use what is available to you.

Summary

Staying fit doesn't require an expensive gym membership or high-end equipment. With creativity, a willingness to try new things and using resources you already have at your disposal, you can create an effective and fulfilling fitness plan. The important thing is that you find enjoyment in exercise and choose activities that you want to maintain long-term. By following these tips, you can lead an active and healthy lifestyle without straining your finances.

Chapter 7: Psychological aspects of weight loss

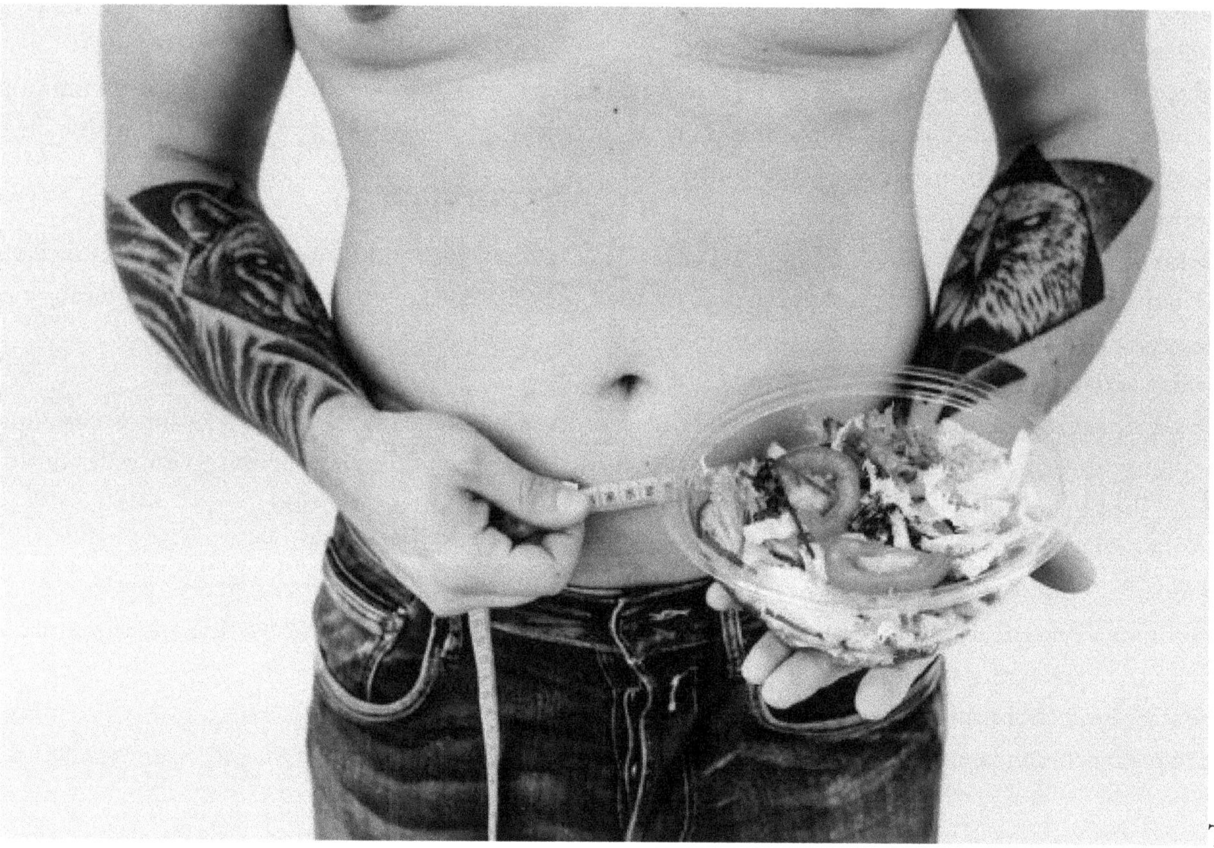

The path to weight loss is not only a physical journey, but also a profoundly psychological one. The mental and emotional challenges that arise along the way can be just as demanding as the physical endeavors. In this chapter, we look at the psychological aspects of weight loss and offer strategies to overcome these mental hurdles and maintain a positive mindset.

The importance of mental attitude

The attitude with which you approach your weight loss can have a decisive influence on your success. A positive, goal-oriented mindset promotes motivation and resilience, while a negative attitude can lead to failure. It is important to set realistic goals and be lenient with yourself to avoid discouragement and self-criticism.

Dealing with self-criticism

Self-criticism is a common obstacle on the road to weight loss. Learn to recognize negative self-talk and replace it with positive affirmations. Remind yourself of your past successes and use them as motivation. See failures as learning opportunities, not as reasons to punish yourself.

The role of support systems

A strong support system can make a huge difference. Share your goals and challenges with family, friends or a support group. Sharing experiences and receiving encouragement from others walking similar paths can help you feel understood and less isolated.

Coping with emotional eating

Many people resort to eating as a coping mechanism in stressful situations or during emotional lows. Identify triggers for emotional eating and develop alternative strategies for coping with stress, such as meditation, walking or creative hobbies. Recognizing and addressing the underlying emotional needs is crucial to breaking this habit.

Self-image and self-worth

Self-image, especially in relation to one's weight, plays an essential role in the psychological dynamics of weight loss. Work on cultivating a healthy self-image that is not solely tied to outward appearances. Appreciate your body for its performance and strength, not just its appearance.

The importance of patience and consistency

Weight loss is a process that takes time. Patience and consistency are crucial to persevere, even if progress seems slow. Set short-term, achievable goals and celebrate every success along the way to keep yourself motivated.

Summary

The psychological aspects of weight loss are multi-layered and complex. Consciously addressing your mental and emotional patterns can help you more effectively manage the challenges that arise along the way. By cultivating a positive attitude, seeking support, addressing emotional eating and promoting a healthy self-image, you will strengthen your mental and emotional resilience. This lays the foundation for lasting success on your weight loss journey.

The role of mental health

Mental health plays a crucial role in the weight loss journey and should not be underestimated. It influences not only our motivation and stamina, but also the way we perceive ourselves and our bodies. In this chapter, we will explore the importance of mental health in the context of weight loss and ways in which you can strengthen your psychological resilience.

Understanding mental health

Mental health encompasses our emotional, psychological and social well-being. It influences how we think, feel and act, particularly in relation to stress, decision making and dealing with challenges. Positive mental health promotes productivity and effectiveness in all areas of life, including weight loss.

The psychological challenges of weight loss

Weight loss is not just a question of physical effort; it is also mentally and emotionally demanding. Self-criticism, discouragement in the face of setbacks and coping with food cravings are just some of the psychological challenges that can occur. In addition, self-image can fluctuate greatly during the weight loss process, which can cause additional emotional stress.

Strategies for strengthening mental health

Develop self-compassion: Be forgiving of yourself and recognize that perfection is unrealistic. Self-compassion promotes resilience and helps you to deal constructively with setbacks.

Cultivate positive self-talk: Pay attention to your inner dialog and replace negative thoughts with positive affirmations. This strengthens your self-esteem and confidence in your own abilities.

Apply stress management techniques: Methods such as deep breathing exercises, meditation or yoga can help to reduce stress and improve mental clarity.

Seek social support: Share your experiences and goals with trusted friends or family members or join a support group. Social support can be a crucial factor in maintaining mental health.

Seek professional help: Don't hesitate to seek professional help if you find that emotional or psychological challenges are hindering your progress. A therapist or psychologist can provide valuable support and strategies.

The link between mental and physical health

Mental and physical health are closely linked. A positive attitude and good mental health can increase motivation for physical activity and healthy eating, while conversely regular exercise and a balanced diet can improve mental health. The result is a synergistic effect that promotes the entire weight loss process.

Summary

Mental health is a fundamental part of the weight loss process and deserves just as much attention and care as physical health. By taking proactive steps to strengthen your mental resilience, you are creating a solid foundation for long-term success and well-being on your weight loss journey. Remember that the path to weight loss is a holistic journey that encompasses both the body and the mind.

Strategies for coping with stress and emotional eating habits

Stress and emotional eating habits are common stumbling blocks on the road to weight loss. Not only can they hinder progress, but they can also lead to a cycle of guilt and self-criticism. Understanding and addressing these behaviors are critical to successful weight loss and fostering a healthy relationship with food. In this chapter, we discuss effective strategies for managing stress and overcoming emotional eating habits.

Recognizing the triggers

The first step to overcoming stress and emotional eating is to recognize the triggers. Often it is specific situations, feelings or people that lead to unhealthy eating habits. Keep a diary to identify patterns and become aware of your triggers.

Development of alternative coping strategies

Once you know your triggers, work on developing alternative strategies for coping with stress that don't involve food. This could include exercise, meditation, deep breathing, keeping a journal or creative hobbies. Find activities that bring you joy and promote relaxation.

Practicing mindfulness

Mindfulness can help you to notice the moment and make more conscious decisions about your eating behavior. Practice mindful eating by taking time to enjoy your meals without distractions and learn to recognize your body's signals of hunger and fullness.

Set realistic goals

Set yourself realistic and achievable goals, both for your diet and for dealing with stress. Unrealistic expectations can lead to frustration and stress, which in turn can trigger emotional eating. Be patient with yourself and recognize that progress takes time.

Seeking social support

Share your challenges and successes with friends, family or a support group. Social support can be a powerful tool for staying motivated and feeling less isolated. Sometimes simply sharing your feelings and experiences can be a relief.

Seek professional help

When stress and emotional eating become overwhelming, don't hesitate to seek professional help. A therapist can offer you individualized strategies and techniques to deal with your specific challenges.

Prioritize self-care

Don't forget to put yourself first and practice regular self-care. Whether it's a relaxing bath, reading a good book or simply spending time in nature, find activities that help you de-stress and look after yourself.

Summary

Managing stress and emotional eating habits takes time, patience and practice. By recognizing your triggers, developing alternative coping strategies and practicing mindfulness, you can build a healthier relationship with food and find a way to manage stress effectively. Remember, every step you take to overcome these challenges is an important contribution to your long-term success and well-being.

Chapter 8: Long-term success strategies

The journey to weight loss and a healthier lifestyle is not a sprint, but a marathon. Long-term success requires not only short-term changes, but also the development and maintenance of habits that can stay with you for a lifetime. In this chapter, we will explore strategies to help you consolidate your successes and stay on track for the long term.

1. focus on sustainability instead of quick fixes

The key to long-term success lies in the sustainability of your lifestyle changes. Quick fixes and extreme diets can provide short-term results, but they are difficult to maintain and often lead to a yo-yo effect. Instead, choose changes that fit into your everyday life and that you can maintain in the long term.

2. make exercise an integral part of your life

Regular physical activity should be a habit that is as natural as brushing your teeth. Find forms of exercise that you enjoy and incorporate them into your daily routine. Whether it's going for a daily walk, cycling, dancing or yoga, the key is to stay active.

3. develop a healthy relationship with food

Food is more than just fuel for the body; it is also a source of pleasure. Instead of seeing food as the enemy, develop a healthy relationship with it. Learn to eat mindfully, enjoy your meals without guilt and listen to your body's signals.

4. remain flexible and adaptable

Life is full of unpredictable events and challenges. Instead of being discouraged by setbacks, see them as opportunities to learn and adapt. Flexibility and the ability to change your strategies when necessary are important for long-term success.

5. set yourself realistic goals

Setting realistic, achievable goals is crucial. They not only provide clear direction, but also measurable milestones to keep you motivated. Celebrate every success, no matter how small, and recognize that progress often comes in small steps.

6. look for social support

Strong support from family, friends or like-minded people can make a big difference. Share your goals and achievements, seek advice and encouragement and offer support yourself. A positive social environment can significantly increase motivation.

7. stay informed and ready to learn

The world of health and fitness is constantly evolving. Stay curious and informed about new research findings, methods and strategies. However, be critical and choose sources that are trustworthy and well-founded.

8. prioritize your well-being

Ultimately, your long-term goal is not just weight loss, but well-being in all areas of your life. Prioritize activities and habits that promote your physical, mental and emotional health.

Summary

Long-term success in weight loss and building a healthier lifestyle requires patience, consistency and a positive attitude. By making sustainable changes, developing a healthy relationship with food and exercise, and seeking support, you are laying the foundation for lasting wellness. Remember that every day is a new opportunity to choose for your health.

How to stay motivated

Motivation is the fuel that drives us forward on our journey to weight loss and a healthier lifestyle. But even the most dedicated people can experience periods when their motivation wanes. The trick is to find ways to renew and maintain that motivation, even when the challenges seem great. In this chapter, we will look at how you can maintain your motivation in the long term.

Remember your "why"

Everyone has a personal reason or reasons for embarking on this journey. Maybe you want to live healthier to be there for your kids, or you have a specific goal weight in mind that is important to you. Keep your "why" present by writing it down and placing it somewhere you can see it every day. This visual reminder can be a powerful motivator.

Celebrate small victories

Weight loss and health improvements are processes that take time. Instead of just focusing on the end goal, celebrate the small successes along the way. Every step in the right direction is a reason to celebrate. Whether it's saying no to an unhealthy snack or reaching a new milestone in exercise, recognize your progress.

Set yourself clear, achievable goals

Big, distant goals can seem overwhelming. Break them down into smaller, specific and achievable goals. Instead of saying, "I want to lose weight," set a goal of, "I want to go for three 30-minute walks this week." This type of goal is measurable and gives you a clear target for the immediate future.

Search for inspiration

Find people, books, podcasts or blogs that inspire and motivate you. Stories of people who have overcome similar challenges can give you new ideas and remind you that your goals are achievable. However, be critical and choose sources that promote healthy and sustainable methods.

Surround yourself with support

A supportive environment can work wonders for your motivation. Whether it's friends, family or an online community - look for people who understand and support your goals. Staying motivated together is often easier than alone.

Learn from setbacks

Setbacks are inevitable, but they are not defeats. See them as learning opportunities and not as a reason to give up. Analyze what went wrong and consider how you can do things differently in the future. The ability to learn from mistakes is a key to long-term success.

Stay flexible

Be ready to adjust your strategies if your circumstances change or if something isn't working. Flexibility in your approach will allow you to stay motivated on the path to weight loss and a healthier lifestyle, even when life is unpredictable.

Summary

Finding and maintaining motivation is a crucial part of your journey. By sticking to your reasons, celebrating small successes, setting clear goals, seeking inspiration, surrounding yourself with support, learning from setbacks and staying flexible, you can keep the flame of motivation burning for the long haul. Remember: every day is a new opportunity to make a choice for your health and well-being.

Making nutrition sustainable

A sustainable diet is not only key to long-term weight loss, but also to maintaining good health and protecting our planet. In this chapter, we focus on how you can adapt your eating habits so that they not only suit you and your goals, but are also feasible and environmentally friendly in the long term.

Understanding what sustainability means

Sustainable eating means choosing food that is healthy for our bodies and at the same time has minimal impact on our environment. It's about finding a balance between what's good for us and what's good for our planet.

Base made from whole, unprocessed foods

The core of a sustainable diet consists of whole, unprocessed foods. Not only are these foods more nutritious, but their production often has a lower environmental impact than that of highly processed foods. Incorporate a variety of fruits, vegetables, whole grains, legumes, nuts and seeds into your daily diet.

Give preference to regional and seasonal products

Buying regional and seasonal produce not only supports the local economy, but also reduces the environmental footprint associated with transporting food over long distances. What's more, seasonal food is often fresher and more nutritious.

Consciously shaping meat consumption

Meat can be part of a sustainable diet if it is consumed consciously. Reduce your meat consumption and, if possible, choose products from animals that have been raised sustainably and in a species-appropriate manner. Think of meat as a side dish rather than the main component of your meals.

Minimize food waste

An important aspect of sustainability is minimizing food waste. Plan your meals in advance, buy only what you need and find creative ways to utilize leftovers. Composting food waste can also help to reduce your ecological footprint.

Pay attention to sustainable packaging

Favor foods with minimal or sustainable packaging to reduce plastic waste. Reusable containers and bags for shopping and storing food are easy ways to minimize your use of single-use plastic.

Making informed decisions

Find out about the origin of your food and the practices of the companies you buy from. Support brands and producers that are committed to sustainable agriculture and fair working conditions.

Summary

Creating a sustainable diet means taking responsibility for your health and the health of our planet. By making conscious choices when shopping and eating, you can not only support your own health goals, but also make a positive contribution to protecting the environment. Remember that every little change counts and the path to a more sustainable diet is a step-by-step process.

The new normal: life after the diet

Once you have reached your target weight, a new phase of your journey begins - life after the diet. This phase is crucial because it's about maintaining the weight you've reached and establishing the new, healthy habits as a permanent part of your life. This chapter focuses on how you can embrace this new normal and be successful in the long term.

Recognize that there is no more "diet"

The first step in the new normal is realizing that the "diet" is now over and a lifelong process of healthy living begins. Instead of thinking of it as a temporary diet, think of your diet and fitness regime as permanent changes. This means incorporating balance and flexibility into your eating habits without falling back into old patterns.

Create a balanced diet

A balanced diet is the key to maintaining your new weight. Instead of maintaining strict bans, learn to enjoy all food groups in moderation. Focus on prioritizing nutrient-rich foods like vegetables, fruits, whole grains, lean protein and healthy fats, while allowing yourself occasional small indulgences.

Develop a routine for regular exercise

Continuing a regular exercise routine is crucial to maintaining your weight and promoting your overall health. Find activities that you enjoy and that can be easily integrated into your daily routine. Be it walking, cycling, yoga or strength training - the goal is to stay active and make exercise a part of your daily life.

Listen to your body

Learn to listen to your body's signals. Eat when you are hungry and stop eating when you are full. Pay attention to your body's reactions to certain foods and adjust your diet accordingly. This mindfulness will help you maintain a healthy relationship with food.

Stay motivated and set yourself new goals

Even after reaching your target weight, it is important to stay motivated and set new goals. These could be fitness goals, health improvements or personal aspirations. Setting and achieving goals promotes a sense of accomplishment and helps to maintain motivation in the long term.

Look for social support

The support of family, friends or like-minded people remains a valuable tool even after the diet. Share your experiences, celebrate your successes and seek advice and support when you face challenges. Strong social support can make the difference between long-term success and falling back into old habits.

Accept that setbacks are normal

Understand that setbacks are part of the process and are not the end of your journey. Cut yourself some slack and realize that perfection is not the goal. Learn from setbacks, adjust your strategies and move on.

Chapter 9: Breakfast recipes

Avocado toast on wholemeal bread

Preparation time: 5 minutes

Cooking time: 2 minutes

Persons: 1

Ingredients:

- 1 slice of wholemeal bread
- 1/2 ripe avocado
- Salt and pepper to taste
- Optional: A pinch of chili flakes or a squeeze of lemon juice

Preparation:

1. **Toasting:** Toast the slice of wholemeal bread in a toaster until it is crispy and golden brown.
2. **Prepare the avocado:** Cut the avocado in half, remove the stone and spoon the flesh from one half into a bowl.
3. **Mash the avocado:** Mash the avocado flesh with a fork to the desired consistency. Season with salt and pepper. Optionally, you can add a squeeze of lemon juice or a pinch of chili flakes to intensify the flavor.
4. **Spread on the bread:** Spread the mashed avocado evenly on the toasted slice of bread.
5. **Serve:** Enjoy your avocado toast immediately while the bread is still warm and crispy.

Macronutrients (estimated):

- Calories: 230 kcal
- Carbohydrates: 26 g
- Protein: 6 g
- Fat: 12 g

Chia pudding with coconut

Preparation time: 5 minutes

Cooking time: 0 minutes (rest overnight or for at least 4 hours)

Persons: 1

Ingredients:

- 3 tablespoons chia seeds
- 200 ml coconut milk (light, for a less calorie-rich option)
- 1/2 teaspoon vanilla extract
- 1 tablespoon maple syrup (or adjust to taste)
- Optional: Fresh fruit or grated coconut for decoration

Preparation:

1. **Mix:** In a medium bowl, whisk together the chia seeds, coconut milk, vanilla extract and maple syrup until well combined.
2. **Leave to rest:** Leave the mixture to stand for about 5 minutes so that the chia seeds can start to absorb the liquid.
3. **Stir and chill:** Stir the mixture again and then cover and place in the fridge. Leave to rest overnight or for at least 4 hours until the pudding has reached a gel-like consistency.
4. **Stir again:** Take the pudding out of the fridge and stir well to make sure the texture is even.
5. **Serve:** Put the chia pudding in a bowl and garnish with fresh fruit or shredded coconut as desired.

Macronutrients (estimated):

- Calories: 300 kcal
- Carbohydrates: 25 g
- Protein: 5 g
- Fat: 20 g

Protein wraps with lean turkey bacon

Preparation time: 10 minutes
Cooking time: 5 minutes
Persons: 1
Ingredients:

- 2 egg whites
- 2 strips of lean turkey bacon
- 1 wholemeal tortilla wrap
- A handful of fresh spinach
- 1 tablespoon low-fat cream cheese
- Salt and pepper to taste
- Optional: A pinch of paprika powder

Preparation:

1. **Fry the turkey bacon:** Fry the turkey bacon in a non-stick frying pan over a medium heat until crispy. After frying, place it on kitchen paper to remove excess fat.
2. **Prepare the egg whites:** Lightly beat the egg whites with salt, pepper and optional paprika powder. Pour them into the same pan and cook over a medium heat until they are firm. Then roll or fold the omelette.
3. **Prepare the wrap:** Spread the wholemeal tortilla evenly with the low-fat cream cheese.
4. **Fill the wrap:** Place the egg white omelette on the wrap, add the crispy turkey bacon and fresh spinach.
5. **Roll the wrap:** Carefully roll up the wrap. If necessary, secure with toothpicks or wrap in parchment paper for easier eating.

Macronutrients (estimated):

- Calories: 250 kcal

- Carbohydrates: 20 g
- Protein: 25 g
- Fat: 8 g

Frittata with vegetables and little fat

Preparation time: 10 minutes

Cooking time: 15 minutes

Persons: 1

Ingredients:

- 2 egg whites and 1 whole egg
- 1/2 cup mixed vegetables (e.g. chopped spinach, peppers, zucchinis)
- 1 tablespoon low-fat milk
- Salt and pepper to taste
- 1 teaspoon olive oil
- Optional: fresh herbs such as basil or parsley for additional flavor

Preparation:

1. **Prepare the vegetables:** Heat the olive oil in a small, ovenproof frying pan over a medium heat. Add the mixed vegetables and fry for a few minutes until soft.
2. **Egg mixture:** In a bowl, beat the egg whites, whole egg and low-fat milk together. Season with salt and pepper. Pour the egg mixture over the sautéed vegetables in the pan.
3. **Cook:** Let the egg and vegetable mixture cook over low to medium heat until the edges are set but the center is still slightly runny, about 5-7 minutes.
4. **Baking:** Place the pan under the grill of your oven and bake the frittata until the top is golden brown and completely set, about 3-5 minutes. Make sure the handle of your pan is ovenproof.
5. **Serve:** Carefully remove the frittata from the pan and serve on a plate. Optionally, you can sprinkle fresh herbs over the finished frittata.

Macronutrients (estimated):

- Calories: 150 kcal
- Carbohydrates: 5 g
- Protein: 15 g
- Fat: 7 g

Boiled eggs and asparagus salad

Preparation time: 10 minutes

Cooking time: 10 minutes

Persons: 1

Ingredients:

- 2 large eggs

- 100g fresh asparagus, ends cut off
- 1 teaspoon extra virgin olive oil
- Salt and pepper to taste
- 1/2 teaspoon Dijon mustard
- 1 tablespoon lemon juice
- Optional: A few leaves of fresh basil or parsley

Preparation:

1. **Boil the eggs:** Place the eggs in a pan of cold water. Bring the water to the boil, then reduce the heat and simmer the eggs for 8-10 minutes for hard-boiled eggs. Then rinse the eggs under cold water and peel.
2. **Cook the asparagus:** Boil the asparagus in a separate pan of lightly salted water for 3-5 minutes until al dente. Then quench in ice water to stop the cooking process and preserve the green color.
3. **Prepare the dressing:** In a small bowl, whisk together the olive oil, lemon juice, Dijon mustard, salt and pepper to make the dressing.
4. **Assemble the salad:** Place the cooled asparagus on a plate, halve the hard-boiled eggs and arrange on top of the asparagus. Drizzle the dressing over the salad.
5. **Garnish with herbs:** Optionally garnish with fresh basil or parsley leaves.

Macronutrients (estimated):

- Calories: approx. 250 kcal
- Carbohydrates: approx. 5 g
- Protein: approx. 13 g
- Fat: approx. 20 g

Roasted chickpeas and avocado salad

Preparation time: 10 minutes
Cooking time: 20 minutes
Persons: 1
Ingredients:

- 1/2 cup chickpeas (from the tin, rinsed and drained)
- 1/2 ripe avocado, diced
- 1 cup mixed leaf lettuce (e.g. rocket, spinach)
- 1 tablespoon of olive oil (for the chickpeas)
- 1/2 teaspoon paprika powder
- Salt and pepper to taste
- 1 tablespoon lemon juice (for the dressing)
- Optional: a handful of chopped cherry tomatoes and/or a small, sliced red onion

Preparation:

1. **Roast the chickpeas:** Preheat your oven to 200°C. Toss the chickpeas with olive oil, paprika powder, salt and

pepper until evenly coated. Spread the chickpeas out on a baking tray and roast for 20 minutes until crispy. Shake the tray occasionally to ensure the chickpeas are roasted evenly.

2. **Prepare the salad:** While the chickpeas are roasting, place the mixed lettuce leaves on a plate.
3. **Add the avocado and other ingredients:** Scatter the diced avocado (and optional cherry tomatoes and red onion) over the lettuce leaves.
4. **Make the dressing:** Drizzle the lemon juice over the salad and season with salt and pepper to taste.
5. **Add the roasted chickpeas:** Remove the roasted chickpeas from the oven and allow them to cool briefly. Then spread them over the salad.

Macronutrients (estimated):

- Calories: 370 kcal
- Carbohydrates: 33 g
- Protein: 12 g
- Fat: 23 g

Greek yogurt with chia seeds and nuts

Preparation time: 5 minutes

Cooking time: 0 minutes

Persons: 1

Ingredients:

- 200g Greek yogurt (low-fat)
- 1 tablespoon chia seeds
- 1 tablespoon of chopped nuts (e.g. almonds, walnuts)
- Optional: a few berries or a teaspoon of honey to sweeten

Preparation:

1. **Prepare the yogurt:** Put the Greek yogurt in a bowl.
2. **Add the chia seeds:** Sprinkle the chia seeds over the yogurt.
3. **Add the nuts:** Add the chopped nuts.
4. **Optional sweetening:** If you like, you can now add a few berries for natural sweetness or a teaspoon of honey.
5. **Mix and serve:** Stir all the ingredients well and leave the yoghurt to stand for a few minutes if necessary so that the chia seeds can swell a little. Then serve.

Macronutrients (estimated):

- Calories: approx. 280 kcal
- Carbohydrates: 19 g
- Protein: 21 g
- Fat: 11 g

Oatmeal with apple and cinnamon

Preparation time: 5 minutes
Cooking time: 5 minutes
Persons: 1
Ingredients:

- 1/2 cup rolled oats (quick cooking)
- 1 cup of water or low-fat milk
- 1 small apple, diced
- 1/2 teaspoon cinnamon
- Optional: 1 teaspoon of honey or maple syrup to sweeten

Preparation:

1. **Cook the oat flakes:** Bring the water or milk to the boil in a small saucepan. Add the rolled oats and reduce the heat. Allow the oats to simmer for about 5 minutes, stirring occasionally, until they are soft.
2. **Add the apple:** Add the diced apples and cinnamon to the oatmeal while it is still cooking. Stir well to ensure the apples soften and the cinnamon is evenly distributed.
3. **Optional sweetener:** If you like, sweeten the oats with a teaspoon of honey or maple syrup.
4. **Serve:** Place the oatmeal mixture in a bowl.
5. **Enjoy:** Enjoy your warm oatmeal with apple and cinnamon.

Macronutrients (estimated):

- Calories: 250 kcal (without honey/maple syrup)
- Carbohydrates: 45 g
- Protein: 10 g
- Fat: 4 g

Pumpkin and oatmeal porridge

Preparation time: 5 minutes
Cooking time: 10 minutes
Persons: 1
Ingredients:

- 1/2 cup rolled oats
- 3/4 cup water or low-fat milk
- 1/4 cup pureed pumpkin (tinned or freshly prepared)
- 1/2 teaspoon cinnamon
- 1 pinch of nutmeg
- 1 pinch of cloves
- Optional: 1 teaspoon of maple syrup or honey to sweeten
- Optional: A handful of chopped nuts or seeds for extra texture

Preparation:

1. **Cook the oats and liquid:** Bring the water or milk to the boil in a small saucepan. Add the oats and reduce the heat. Leave to simmer for about 5 minutes, stirring occasionally.
2. **Stir in the pumpkin puree:** Add the pumpkin puree and spices (cinnamon, nutmeg, cloves) to the oats. Stir everything well so that the flavors combine.
3. **Optional sweetener:** If you like, sweeten your porridge with maple syrup or honey.
4. **Additional ingredients:** Add chopped nuts or seeds, if desired, to give the porridge a crunchy texture.
5. **Serve:** Put the finished porridge in a bowl and enjoy it warm.

Macronutrients (estimated):

- Calories: 220 kcal (depending on the selected ingredients and sweeteners)
- Carbohydrates: 40 g
- Protein: 10 g
- Fat: 7 g (depending on whether nuts or seeds are added)

Lentil and spinach breakfast pans

Preparation time: 5 minutes
Cooking time: 10 minutes
Persons: 1
Ingredients:

- 1/2 cup pre-cooked lentils (from the tin, rinsed and drained)
- 1 handful of fresh spinach
- 1 small egg
- 1 teaspoon olive oil
- Salt and pepper to taste
- Optional: a pinch of paprika powder or chili flakes for a little spiciness
- Optional: a tablespoon of low-fat yogurt or a squeeze of lemon juice to serve

Preparation:

1. **Prepare the spinach:** Heat the olive oil in a small frying pan over a medium heat. Add the spinach and sauté until wilted, about 1-2 minutes.
2. **Add the lentils:** Add the rinsed lentils to the spinach in the pan. Season with salt, pepper and optional paprika powder or chili flakes. Fry the mixture for a further 2-3 minutes until well heated.
3. **Fry the egg:** Make a small well in the center of the lentil and spinach mixture and crack the egg into it. Cover the pan and cook the egg for 3-5 minutes until the egg white is set but the yolk is still slightly runny.
4. **Finish:** Check that the egg is cooked to your liking and remove the pan from the heat.
5. **Serve:** Place the lentil, spinach and egg mixture on a plate. Optionally, you can add a tablespoon of low-fat yogurt or a squeeze of lemon juice on top.

Macronutrients (estimated):

- Calories: 275kcal
- Carbohydrates: 23 g
- Protein: 18 g
- Fat: 11 g

Lean chicken sausage and vegetable pan

Preparation time: 5 minutes

Cooking time: 10 minutes

Persons: 1

Ingredients:

- 2 lean chicken sausages, cut into slices
- 1/2 cup broccoli, cut into florets
- 1/2 red bell pepper, diced
- 1/2 yellow zucchini, cut into slices
- 1 teaspoon olive oil
- Salt and pepper to taste
- Optional: A pinch of chili flakes or Italian herbs for extra flavor

Preparation:

1. **Prepare the vegetables:** Heat the olive oil in a medium frying pan over a medium heat. Add the broccoli, red bell pepper and yellow zucchini. Sauté the vegetables for about 5 minutes, stirring occasionally, until slightly softened.
2. **Add the chicken sausage:** Add the sliced chicken sausages to the vegetables in the pan. Season with salt, pepper and optional chili flakes or Italian herbs. Cook everything together for a further 5 minutes until the sausages are cooked through and the vegetables are tender.
3. **Mix well: Make** sure that the sausage slices and vegetables are well mixed together and have been cooked all the way through.
4. **Scason to taste:** Taste the vegetable pan and adjust the seasoning if necessary.
5. **Serve:** Transfer the chicken sausage and vegetable skillet to a plate and enjoy hot.

Macronutrients (estimated):

- Calorics: 330 kcal
- Carbohydrates: 11 g
- Protein: 27 g
- Fat: 16 g

Muesli with low-fat milk and fresh fruit

Preparation time: 5 minutes

Cooking time: 0 minutes

Persons: 1

Ingredients:

- 1/2 cup muesli (no added sugar)
- 3/4 cup low-fat milk
- 1/2 cup fresh fruit of your choice (e.g. berries, apple pieces, banana slices)
- Optional: 1 teaspoon of honey or maple syrup for extra sweetness
- Optional: A tablespoon of chopped nuts or seeds for more texture and nutrients

Preparation:

1. **Prepare the muesli:** Put the muesli in a bowl.
2. **Add milk:** Pour the low-fat milk over the muesli.
3. **Add the fruit:** Add the fresh fruit of your choice.
4. **Optionally sweeten and garnish:** If you like, sweeten the muesli with a teaspoon of honey or maple syrup and/or garnish with chopped nuts or seeds.
5. **Serve:** Stir and enjoy immediately.

Macronutrients (estimated):

- Calories: 260 kcal
- Carbohydrates: 47 g
- Protein: 12 g
- Fat: 5 g (depending on whether nuts or seeds are added)

Omelette with spinach and feta

Preparation time: 5 minutes
Cooking time: 5 minutes
Persons: 1
Ingredients:

- 2 large eggs
- 1/2 cup fresh spinach, roughly chopped
- 30g feta cheese, crumbled
- 1 teaspoon olive oil
- Salt and pepper to taste

Preparation:

1. **Beat the eggs:** Break the eggs into a bowl and season with salt and pepper. Whisk well until the mixture is uniform.
2. **Sauté the spinach:** Heat the olive oil in a small frying pan over a medium heat. Add the spinach and sauté briefly until it collapses, about 1-2 minutes.
3. **Add the eggs:** Pour the beaten eggs over the spinach in the pan. Move the pan slightly to distribute the egg mixture evenly.
4. **Add the feta:** Sprinkle the crumbled feta over the omelette while the underside is cooking but the top is still slightly runny.

5. **Fold the omelette:** Fold the omelette in half when the underside is firm and the top is still slightly moist. Leave it in the pan for another 1 minute to warm through.

Macronutrients (estimated):

- Calories: 310 kcal
- Carbohydrates: 2g
- Protein: 22 g
- Fat: 25 g

Wholemeal buttermilk pancakes

Preparation time: 10 minutes
Cooking time: 10 minutes
Persons: 1
Ingredients:

- 1/2 cup wholemeal flour
- 1/2 cup buttermilk (low-fat)
- 1 large egg
- 1/2 teaspoon baking powder
- 1 pinch of salt
- 1 teaspoon honey or maple syrup
- 1/2 teaspoon vanilla extract
- 1 teaspoon of olive oil or another neutral oil for the pan

Preparation:

1. **Prepare the dough:** In a medium bowl, mix together the whole wheat flour, baking powder and salt. In another bowl, whisk together the egg, buttermilk, honey (or maple syrup) and vanilla extract until well combined. Add the wet ingredients to the dry ingredients and stir until just combined.
2. **Heat the pan:** Heat the olive oil in a non-stick frying pan over a medium heat.
3. **Cook the pancakes:** Add about 1/4 cup batter per pancake to the pan. Cook each pancake until small bubbles appear on the surface and the edges look firm, then flip and cook on the other side until golden brown.
4. **Repeat:** Repeat the process with the remaining dough.
5. **Serve:** Serve the pancakes warm with a topping of your choice, such as fresh fruit or a dollop of yogurt.

Macronutrients (estimated):

- Calories: 370 kcal
- Carbohydrates: 53 g
- Protein: 15 g
- Fat: 11 g

Protein smoothie with spinach and berries

Preparation time: 5 minutes

Cooking time: 0 minutes

Persons: 1

Ingredients:

- 1 cup fresh spinach
- 1/2 cup frozen mixed berries (e.g. strawberries, blueberries, raspberries)
- 1/2 banana
- 1/2 cup low-fat milk or a plant-based alternative
- 1 measuring spoon of protein powder (preferably unflavored or vanilla)
- Optional: 1 teaspoon of chia seeds or linseed for extra fiber and omega-3 fatty acids

Preparation:

1. **Prepare the ingredients:** Wash the spinach thoroughly and cut the banana into pieces.
2. **Mix all the ingredients:** Place the spinach, frozen berries, banana, protein powder and milk (or plant-based alternative) in a blender.
3. **Add optional ingredients:** If you like, add the chia seeds or linseed now.
4. **Blend:** Blend all ingredients on high speed until the smoothie is smooth and creamy.
5. **Serve:** Pour the smoothie into a glass and enjoy immediately.

Macronutrients (estimated):

- Calories: 275 kcal
- Carbohydrates: 33 g
- Protein: 22 g
- Fat: 4 g

Quinoa breakfast bowl with berries

Preparation time: 5 minutes (if quinoa is already cooked)

Cooking time: 15 minutes (for the quinoa, if not already pre-cooked)

Persons: 1

Ingredients:

- 1/2 cup cooked quinoa
- 1/2 cup low-fat milk or a plant-based milk alternative
- 1/2 cup fresh berries (e.g. strawberries, blueberries, raspberries)
- 1 tablespoon of chopped nuts (e.g. walnuts, almonds)
- Optional: 1 teaspoon of honey or maple syrup to sweeten
- Optional: A pinch of cinnamon for extra flavor

Preparation:

1. **Cook quinoa:** If the quinoa is not precooked, rinse 1/4 cup uncooked quinoa and boil it with 1/2 cup water. Bring to a boil, then reduce the heat and simmer for 15 minutes until the water is absorbed.
2. **Reheat the quinoa:** Heat the cooked quinoa with the milk in a small saucepan over a medium heat until hot.
3. **Prepare the berries:** While the quinoa is heating, wash the berries and cut larger pieces as needed.
4. **Assemble the bowl:** Pour the warm quinoa and milk mixture into a bowl. Add the fresh berries and chopped nuts.
5. **Optional sweetening and seasoning:** Sweeten your breakfast bowl with honey or maple syrup and add a pinch of cinnamon to taste.

Macronutrients (estimated):

- Calories: 310 kcal
- Carbohydrates: 47 g
- Protein: 12 g
- Fat: 8 g

Sweet potato and black bean burritos

Preparation time: 10 minutes
Cooking time: 20 minutes
Persons: 1
Ingredients:

- 1 small sweet potato, diced
- 1/2 cup black beans (from the tin, rinsed and drained)
- 1 wholemeal tortilla wrap
- 1/4 cup grated cheese (low-fat)
- 2 tablespoons salsa
- 1 tablespoon olive oil
- 1/2 teaspoon cumin
- Salt and pepper to taste
- Optional: fresh coriander, chopped

Preparation:

1. **Cook the sweet potatoes:** Heat the olive oil in a frying pan over a medium heat. Add the diced sweet potatoes, season with cumin, salt and pepper. Roast the sweet potatoes until they are soft, about 15-20 minutes.
2. **Add the beans:** Add the black beans to the sweet potatoes in the pan. Cook everything together for a further 5 minutes.
3. **Prepare the wrap:** Heat the whole wheat tortilla wrap in another skillet or in the oven until warm and flexible.
4. **Fill the burrito:** Spread the sweet potato and bean mixture in the center of the wrap, add salsa and shredded cheese. Optionally, you can add fresh cilantro for extra flavor.
5. **Roll the burrito:** Fold in the sides of the wrap and roll it up tightly. Optionally, you can fry the burrito in a pan on both sides to make it crispy.

Macronutrients (estimated):

- Calories: 440 kcal
- Carbohydrates: 63 g
- Protein: 17 g
- Fat: 18 g

Tofu scramble with vegetables

Preparation time: 5 minutes
Cooking time: 10 minutes
Persons: 1
Ingredients:

- 1/2 block of firm tofu, well drained and crumbled
- 1/4 cup chopped onion
- 1/2 cup mixed vegetables (e.g. peppers, spinach, tomatoes)
- 1 tablespoon olive oil
- 1/2 teaspoon turmeric (for the color)
- Salt and pepper to taste
- Optional: 1/4 teaspoon smoked paprika or chili flakes for some spice
- Optional: Fresh herbs for garnish (e.g. parsley or coriander)

Preparation:

1. **Sauté the vegetables:** Heat the olive oil in a frying pan over a medium heat. Add the chopped onion and fry until softened. Then add the rest of the vegetables and fry until slightly soft.
2. **Add the tofu:** Add the crumbled tofu to the vegetable mixture in the pan. Sprinkle everything with turmeric, salt and pepper (and optionally smoked paprika or chili flakes).
3. **Cook scramble:** Cook the mixture, stirring occasionally, until the tofu is hot and the seasonings are evenly distributed, about 5-7 minutes.
4. **Seasoning:** Taste the tofu scramble and adjust the seasoning if necessary.
5. **Serve:** Transfer the tofu scramble to a plate and optionally garnish with fresh herbs.

Macronutrients (estimated):

- Calories: 220 kcal
- Carbohydrates: 12 g
- Protein: 17 g
- Fat: 13 g

Zucchini muffins (sugar-free)

Preparation time: 10 minutes
Cooking time: 20 minutes
Persons: 1

Ingredients:

- 1/4 cup wholemeal flour
- 1/4 cup ground almonds
- 1/2 small zucchini, grated
- 1 large egg
- 1 tablespoon unsweetened apple sauce
- 1/2 teaspoon baking powder
- 1 pinch of salt
- 1/2 teaspoon cinnamon
- Optional: nuts or seeds for extra texture

Preparation:

1. **Preheat the oven:** Preheat the oven to 180°C and grease two muffin tins or use muffin paper cases.
2. **Mix the dry ingredients:** In a bowl, mix together the wholemeal flour, ground almonds, baking powder, salt and cinnamon.
3. **Add the wet ingredients:** Beat the egg in a separate bowl and mix with the unsweetened applesauce and grated zucchini. Add the wet ingredients to the dry ingredients and stir until well combined. Add optional nuts or seeds.
4. **Spread the batter:** Divide the batter evenly between the prepared muffin tins.
5. **Bake:** Bake muffins for 20 minutes or until a toothpick comes out clean.

Macronutrients (estimated per muffin, for 2 muffins):

- Calories: 175 kcal
- Carbohydrates: 20 g
- Protein: 8 g
- Fat: 10 g

Chapter 10: Recipes for lunch

Eggplant lasagna with ricotta and spinach

Preparation time: 15 minutes

Cooking time: 30 minutes

Persons: 1

Ingredients:

- 1 large eggplant, cut into long slices
- 100g ricotta (low-fat)
- 1/2 cup fresh spinach, roughly chopped
- 1/4 cup strained tomatoes
- 1 clove of garlic, finely chopped
- 1 tablespoon olive oil
- Salt and pepper to taste
- 1/4 teaspoon dried oregano
- 30g grated mozzarella (low-fat)

Preparation:

1. **Prepare the eggplant:** Preheat the oven to 200°C. Brush both sides of the eggplant slices lightly with olive oil and place them on a baking tray lined with baking paper. Bake for 10-15 minutes or until soft.
2. **Mix the filling:** While the eggplant is in the oven, mix the ricotta, spinach, garlic, salt, pepper and oregano in a bowl.
3. **Layers:** Take a small oven dish and spread a thin layer of the tomato puree on the bottom. Place a layer of the baked eggplant slices on top, followed by a layer of the ricotta and spinach mixture. Repeat the layers until all the ingredients are used up, finishing with a layer of the tomato puree.
4. **Bake:** Sprinkle the top layer with the grated mozzarella. Bake the lasagne in the oven for a further 15-20 minutes until the cheese is melted and lightly browned.
5. **Serve:** Leave the lasagna to cool for a few minutes before serving.

Macronutrients (estimated):

- Calories: 375 kcal
- Carbohydrates: 22 g
- Protein: 20 g
- Fat: 20 g

Cauliflower rice with chicken and vegetables

Preparation time: 10 minutes

Cooking time: 15 minutes

Persons: 1

Ingredients:

- 1/2 head of cauliflower, cut into florets and processed into "rice"
- 100g chicken breast, cut into cubes
- 1/2 cup broccoli, cut into small florets
- 1/2 carrot, cut into thin strips
- 1/4 onion, finely diced
- 1 clove of garlic, finely chopped
- 1 tablespoon olive oil
- Salt and pepper to taste
- Optional: soy sauce or tamari for extra flavor

Preparation:

1. **Prepare the cauliflower: Process** the cauliflower florets in a food processor until they have the consistency of rice.
2. **Fry the chicken:** Heat a tablespoon of olive oil in a frying pan and fry the chicken breast cubes until they are fully cooked. Remove them from the pan and set aside.
3. **Cook the vegetables:** Add the onion and garlic to the same pan and sauté until soft. Then add the broccoli and carrots and cook until the vegetables are al dente.
4. **Add the cauliflower rice: Add** the cauliflower rice to the vegetable mixture, season with salt and pepper (and optional soy sauce or tamari) and cook everything together for about 5 minutes.
5. **Add the chicken again:** Return the fried chicken breast cubes to the pan and mix well until the ingredients are evenly heated.

Macronutrients (estimated):

- Calories: 330 kcal
- Carbohydrates: 17 g
- Protein: 33 g
- Fat: 12 g

Broccoli quiche without base

Preparation time: 10 minutes
Cooking time: 25 minutes
Persons: 1
Ingredients:

- 1 cup fresh broccoli, cut into small florets
- 2 large eggs
- 1/4 cup milk (low-fat)
- 30g grated cheese (low-fat, e.g. Cheddar or Gouda)
- 1/4 teaspoon salt
- 1/4 teaspoon black pepper
- 1/4 teaspoon nutmeg
- Optional: 1 tablespoon finely chopped onion for extra flavor

Preparation:

1. **Preheat the oven:** Preheat the oven to 180°C.
2. **Prepare the broccoli:** Blanch the broccoli in boiling water for 2-3 minutes until slightly soft but still has a bite. Drain and set aside.
3. **Egg and milk mixture:** In a bowl, whisk together the eggs, milk, salt, pepper and nutmeg. Add the grated cheese and mix well.
4. **Assemble the quiche:** Place the blanched broccoli (and optional chopped onion) evenly in a small baking dish lined with baking paper or greased. Pour the egg, milk and cheese mixture over the top.
5. **Bake:** Bake the quiche in the preheated oven for 25 minutes, or until the egg mixture is set and the top is lightly browned.

Macronutrients (estimated):

- Calories: 275 kcal
- Carbohydrates: 8 g
- Protein: 22 g
- Fat: 17 g

Colorful lentil salad with feta and fresh herbs

Preparation time: 10 minutes
Cooking time: 20 minutes (if the lentils are not pre-cooked)
Persons: 1
Ingredients:

- 1/2 cup lentils (preferably a colorful mixture)
- 2 cups of water (for cooking the lentils)
- 1/4 cup feta cheese, crumbled
- 1/2 cup cherry tomatoes, halved
- 1/4 cup cucumber, diced
- 1/4 cup red bell pepper, diced
- 1/4 cup fresh herbs (e.g. parsley, mint), roughly chopped
- 1 tablespoon olive oil
- 1 tablespoon lemon juice
- Salt and pepper to taste

Preparation:

1. **Cook the lentils:** Rinse the lentils and cook them in 2 cups of water until they are soft but still have a bite, about 20 minutes. Then drain and leave to cool.
2. **Prepare the vegetables and herbs:** While the lentils are cooking, prepare the cherry tomatoes, cucumber, red bell pepper and fresh herbs.
3. **Mix the dressing:** In a small bowl, whisk together olive oil, lemon juice, salt and pepper to make the dressing.
4. **Assemble the salad:** In a large bowl, mix the cooled lentils with the tomatoes, cucumber, peppers and herbs.

Add the crumbled feta.

5. **Mix with dressing:** Pour the dressing over the salad and mix everything well.

Macronutrients (estimated):

- Calories: 375 kcal
- Carbohydrates: 43 g
- Protein: 20 g
- Fat: 17 g

Mushroom and spinach omelette

Preparation time: 5 minutes
Cooking time: 10 minutes
Persons: 1
Ingredients:

- 2 large eggs
- 1/2 cup fresh mushrooms, sliced
- 1/2 cup fresh spinach, roughly chopped
- 1 tablespoon low-fat milk
- 1 teaspoon olive oil
- Salt and pepper to taste
- Optional: 1 tablespoon grated cheese (low-fat)

Preparation:

1. **Prepare the eggs:** Beat the eggs with the low-fat milk in a bowl. Season the mixture with salt and pepper.
2. **Sauté the vegetables:** Heat the olive oil in a frying pan over a medium heat. Add the mushrooms and fry until soft. Then add the spinach and fry until it collapses.
3. **Add the eggs:** Pour the egg and milk mixture over the vegetables in the pan. Move the pan slightly to distribute the eggs evenly.
4. **Optionally, add cheese:** If you are using cheese, sprinkle it over the top of the omelette while it is still liquid.
5. **Finish the omelette:** Fold the omelette in half when the underside is firm and the top is still slightly moist. Leave it in the pan for another 1-2 minutes to warm through.

Macronutrients (estimated):

- Calories: 225 kcal
- Carbohydrates: 4 g
- Protein: 15 g
- Fat: 16 g

Fried tofu with zucchini noodles

Preparation time: 10 minutes

Cooking time: 10 minutes
Persons: 1
Ingredients:

- 100g firm tofu, drained and cut into cubes
- 1 medium-sized zucchini, spiralized or cut into thin strips
- 1 teaspoon olive oil
- 1 clove of garlic, finely chopped
- Salt and pepper to taste
- Optional: 1 tablespoon of soy sauce or tamari
- Optional: a few chili flakes for extra spiciness
- Optional: Fresh herbs such as basil or parsley to garnish

Preparation:

1. **Fry the tofu:** Heat the olive oil in a frying pan over a medium heat. Add the tofu and fry until golden brown on all sides, about 5-7 minutes. Optionally, you can add soy sauce or tamari while frying to give the tofu more flavor.
2. **Add the garlic:** Add the chopped garlic to the pan and sauté briefly with the tofu to make it aromatic. Make sure that the garlic does not burn.
3. **Prepare the zucchini noodles:** In another pan, sauté the zucchini noodles with a little olive oil over a medium heat for 2-3 minutes until they are slightly soft but still have a bite. Season with salt and pepper.
4. **Combine: Add** the fried tofu cubes to the zucchini noodles in the pan and mix everything well. Optionally, you can now add chili flakes if you like it spicier.
5. **Serve:** Transfer the mixture to a plate and garnish with fresh herbs, if using.

Macronutrients (estimated):

- Calories: 280 kcal
- Carbohydrates: 12 g
- Protein: 18 g
- Fat: 16 g

Stuffed peppers with quinoa and vegetables

Preparation time: 15 minutes
Cooking time: 30 minutes
Persons: 1
Ingredients:

- 1 large red bell pepper, halved and deseeded
- 1/4 cup quinoa, uncooked
- 1/2 cup vegetable stock (for cooking the quinoa)
- 1/4 cup zucchini, diced
- 1/4 cup tomatoes, diced

- 1/4 cup black beans, rinsed and drained
- 1 tablespoon olive oil
- Salt and pepper to taste
- 1/4 teaspoon cumin
- 2 tablespoons grated cheese (optional, low-fat)

Preparation:

1. **Cook the quinoa:** Cook the quinoa in the vegetable stock according to the packet instructions until it is soft and has absorbed the liquid.
2. **Prepare the vegetables:** While the quinoa is cooking, heat the olive oil in a pan. Add the zucchini and tomatoes, season with salt, pepper and cumin and fry for about 5 minutes until the vegetables are soft.
3. **Quinoa and vegetable mixture:** Add the cooked quinoa and black beans to the vegetables in the pan and mix well.
4. **Stuff the peppers:** Fill the bell pepper halves with the quinoa and vegetable mixture and place in an ovenproof dish. Optionally, sprinkle with grated cheese.
5. **Bake:** Bake the stuffed peppers at 180°C for about 20 minutes until the peppers are soft and the cheese has melted.

Macronutrients (estimated):

- Calories: 385 kcal
- Carbohydrates: 47 g
- Protein: 14 g
- Fat: 13 g

Vegetable broth with chicken strips

Preparation time: 10 minutes
Cooking time: 20 minutes
Persons: 1
Ingredients:

- 150g chicken breast, cut into strips
- 2 cups vegetable stock (low sodium)
- 1/2 carrot, cut into thin slices
- 1/2 stalk celery, finely chopped
- 1/4 onion, finely diced
- 1/4 cup frozen peas
- 1 teaspoon olive oil
- Salt and pepper to taste
- Optional: fresh herbs such as parsley or thyme to garnish

Preparation:

1. **Brown the chicken:** Heat the olive oil in a saucepan over a medium heat. Add the chicken strips, season with salt and pepper and fry until lightly browned all over.
2. **Sauté the vegetables:** Add the onion, carrot and celery to the chicken in the pan. Sauté everything for about 5 minutes until the vegetables are soft.
3. **Add the stock:** Pour the vegetable stock into the pan and bring the mixture to the boil. Then reduce the heat and allow the soup to simmer for about 10 minutes.
4. **Add the peas:** Add the frozen peas and cook the soup for a further 5 minutes until the peas are warm.
5. **Serve:** Taste the soup and adjust the seasoning as required. Serve the vegetable broth with chicken strips hot, garnished with fresh herbs, if using.

Macronutrients (estimated):

- Calories: 275 kcal
- Carbohydrates: 12 g
- Protein: 33 g
- Fat: 8 g

Vegetable pan with prawns

Preparation time: 10 minutes
Cooking time: 10 minutes
Persons: 1
Ingredients:

- 100g prawns, peeled and deveined
- 1/2 cup broccoli, cut into small florets
- 1/2 cup paprika, cut into strips
- 1/4 cup zucchini, cut into half moons
- 1/4 cup carrots, cut into thin slices
- 1 clove of garlic, finely chopped
- 1 tablespoon olive oil
- Salt and pepper to taste
- Optional: 1 teaspoon of soy sauce or tamari for extra flavor
- Optional: chili flakes or fresh lemon juice to taste

Preparation:

1. **Prepare the vegetables:** Heat the olive oil in a large frying pan or wok over a medium heat. Add the chopped garlic and sauté briefly until fragrant.
2. **Sauté the vegetables:** Add the carrots and broccoli to the pan and fry for approx. 3-4 minutes. Then add the peppers and zucchinis and fry for a further 3-4 minutes until the vegetables are al dente.
3. **Add the prawns:** Add the prawns to the vegetables in the pan. Season with salt, pepper and optional soy sauce or tamari. Fry the prawns until they are cooked through and pink in color, about 2-3 minutes.
4. **Season to taste:** Taste the dish and add additional spices if necessary, such as chili flakes or a squeeze of fresh lemon juice.

5. **Serve:** Serve the vegetable pan with prawns immediately while it is still hot.

Macronutrients (estimated):

- Calories: 280 kcal
- Carbohydrates: 12 g
- Protein: 22 g
- Fat: 13 g

Cucumber and tomato salad with cottage cheese

Preparation time: 5 minutes
Cooking time: 0 minutes
Persons: 1
Ingredients:

- 1/2 large cucumber, cut into slices
- 1/2 cup cherry tomatoes, halved
- 1/2 cup cottage cheese (low-fat)
- 1 tablespoon olive oil
- 1 tablespoon lemon juice
- Salt and pepper to taste
- Optional: fresh herbs such as dill or parsley, chopped

Preparation:

1. **Prepare the cucumber and tomatoes:** Wash the cucumber and cherry tomatoes thoroughly. Cut the cucumber into thin slices and halve the tomatoes.
2. **Serve the salad:** Arrange the cucumber slices and tomato halves on a plate.
3. **Add the cottage cheese:** Spoon the cottage cheese over the vegetables.
4. **Prepare the dressing:** In a small bowl, mix the olive oil with the lemon juice. Season the dressing with salt and pepper. Pour the dressing evenly over the salad.
5. **Add optional herbs:** Sprinkle the salad with fresh herbs, if using.

Macronutrients (estimated):

- Calories: 225 kcal
- Carbohydrates: 12 g
- Protein: 18 g
- Fat: 13 g

Chicken breast on rocket with balsamic dressing

Preparation time: 10 minutes
Cooking time: 15 minutes
Persons: 1

Ingredients:

- 1 chicken breast (approx. 150g)
- 2 cups rocket
- 1/2 cup cherry tomatoes, halved
- 1 tablespoon of olive oil (for the chicken)
- Salt and pepper to taste
- 1 tablespoon balsamic vinegar
- 1 teaspoon Dijon mustard
- 1 teaspoon honey
- 2 tablespoons of olive oil (for the dressing)

Preparation:

1. **Prepare the chicken breast:** Season the chicken breast with salt and pepper and fry in a pan with 1 tablespoon of olive oil over a medium heat for about 7 minutes on each side until cooked through. Remove from the pan and leave to rest.
2. **Prepare the dressing:** In a small bowl, whisk together the balsamic vinegar, Dijon mustard, honey and 2 tablespoons of olive oil to make the dressing. Season to taste with salt and pepper.
3. **Serve the salad:** Arrange the rocket and halved cherry tomatoes on a plate.
4. **Serve the chicken breast:** Cut the rested chicken breast into thin slices and arrange on the rocket.
5. **Serve with dressing:** Drizzle the balsamic dressing over the chicken breast and rocket.

Macronutrients (estimated):

- Calories: 375 kcal
- Carbohydrates: 12 g
- Protein: 27 g
- Fat: 22 g

Cod fillet with broccoli and almonds

Preparation time: 10 minutes
Cooking time: 20 minutes
Persons: 1
Ingredients:

- 1 cod fillet (approx. 150g)
- 1 cup broccoli florets
- 1 tablespoon of slivered almonds
- 1 tablespoon olive oil
- Salt and pepper to taste
- Optional: lemon slices for garnish

Preparation:

1. **Preheat the oven:** Preheat the oven to 200°C.
2. **Prepare the broccoli: Spread** the broccoli florets on a baking tray lined with baking paper. Drizzle with a little olive oil and season with salt and pepper. Bake in the preheated oven for about 10 minutes until almost cooked.
3. **Prepare the cod:** Place the cod fillet on the baking tray with the broccoli florets. Drizzle the fillet with the remaining olive oil and season with salt and pepper.
4. **Bake: Sprinkle the** almond slivers over the broccoli and cod fillet. Place the baking tray back in the oven and bake for a further 10 minutes, or until the fish is fully cooked and the almonds are lightly toasted.
5. **Serve:** Serve the cod fillet and broccoli hot, garnished with fresh lemon slices, if desired.

Macronutrients (estimated):

- Calories: 335 kcal
- Carbohydrates: 8 g
- Protein: 30 g
- Fat: 16 g

Carrot and ginger soup

Preparation time: 10 minutes

Cooking time: 20 minutes

Persons: 1

Ingredients:

- 3 large carrots, peeled and roughly chopped
- 1 small piece of ginger, peeled and finely chopped (approx. 1 teaspoon)
- 1/2 onion, finely diced
- 1 clove of garlic, finely chopped
- 2 cups vegetable stock
- 1 tablespoon olive oil
- Salt and pepper to taste
- Optional: 1 tablespoon of coconut milk or cream to garnish

Preparation:

1. **Sauté the vegetables:** Heat the olive oil in a saucepan over a medium heat. Add the onion, garlic and ginger and sauté until the onion is translucent.
2. **Add the carrots:** Add the chopped carrots to the pot and cook for a few minutes until they soften slightly.
3. **Cook the soup:** Pour the vegetable stock into the pan, increase the heat and bring the soup to the boil. Then reduce the heat and allow the soup to simmer for 15-20 minutes until the carrots are soft.
4. **Puree the soup:** Remove the pan from the heat and puree the soup with a hand blender or in a blender until smooth. Season with salt and pepper.
5. **Serve:** Serve the soup hot, garnished with a tablespoon of coconut milk or cream, if using.

Macronutrients (estimated):

- Calories: 225 kcal
- Carbohydrates: 21 g
- Protein: 4 g
- Fat: 8 g

Chickpea salad with peppers and onions

Preparation time: 10 minutes
Cooking time: 0 minutes
Persons: 1
Ingredients:

- 1/2 cup chickpeas (precooked or canned, rinsed and drained)
- 1/2 red bell pepper, cut into cubes
- 1/4 red onion, finely chopped
- 1 tablespoon olive oil
- 1 tablespoon fresh lemon juice
- Salt and pepper to taste
- Optional: fresh herbs such as parsley or coriander, chopped

Preparation:

1. **Prepare the ingredients:** If you are using tinned chickpeas, rinse them thoroughly under cold water and drain. Cut the peppers into cubes and finely chop the red onion.
2. **Mix the salad:** In a bowl, mix the drained chickpeas with the diced peppers and chopped onion.
3. **Mix the dressing:** In a small bowl, mix the olive oil with the fresh lemon juice. Season to taste with salt and pepper.
4. **Dress the salad: Pour** the dressing over the chickpea salad and mix everything well. Leave the salad to stand briefly so that the flavors can develop.
5. **Serve:** Optionally garnish the salad with fresh herbs before serving.

Macronutrients (estimated):

- Calories: 280 kcal
- Carbohydrates: 33 g
- Protein: 12 g
- Fat: approx. 10-15 g

Salmon fillet with asparagus and lemon butter

Preparation time: 10 minutes
Cooking time: 15 minutes
Persons: 1
Ingredients:

- 1 salmon fillet (approx. 150g)

- 1/2 bunch fresh asparagus, ends cut
- 1 tablespoon butter (reduced-fat, if preferred)
- 1/2 lemon, juice and zest
- Salt and pepper to taste
- Optional: fresh herbs such as dill or parsley

Preparation:

1. **Preheat the oven:** Preheat the oven to 200°C.
2. **Prepare the salmon and asparagus:** Place the salmon fillet and asparagus next to each other on a baking tray lined with baking paper. Drizzle a little olive oil over the asparagus and season both with salt and pepper.
3. **Bake:** Place the baking tray in the oven and bake for about 12-15 minutes, or until the salmon is cooked through and the asparagus is tender.
4. **Prepare the lemon butter:** While the salmon and asparagus are in the oven, melt the butter in a small saucepan and mix in the lemon juice and zest. Optionally, you can add fresh herbs for extra flavor.
5. **Serve:** Place the salmon fillet and asparagus on a plate and pour the lemon butter over both. Serve immediately.

Macronutrients (estimated):

- Calories: 333 kcal
- Carbohydrates: 8 g
- Protein: 23 g
- Fat: 22 g

Mediterranean vegetable casserole

Preparation time: 15 minutes
Cooking time: 30 minutes
Persons: 1
Ingredients:

- 1/2 zucchini, sliced
- 1/2 eggplant, sliced
- 1/2 red bell pepper, cut into strips
- 1/2 yellow bell pepper, cut into strips
- 1 tomato, sliced
- 1 clove of garlic, finely chopped
- 2 tablespoons olive oil
- 1 teaspoon dried oregano
- Salt and pepper to taste
- 2 tablespoons grated Parmesan (optional)

Preparation:

1. **Preheat the oven:** Preheat the oven to 180°C.

2. **Prepare the vegetables:** In a large bowl, mix the zucchini, eggplant, bell pepper, tomato and garlic with the olive oil, oregano, salt and pepper.
3. **Layers:** Layer the vegetables in a small, ovenproof dish. Alternate the vegetables to create a colorful mixture.
4. **Bake:** Cover the dish with aluminum foil and bake the vegetables for about 20 minutes. Then remove the foil, optionally sprinkle with Parmesan cheese and bake for a further 10 minutes until the vegetables are soft and the cheese has melted.
5. **Serve:** Allow the casserole to cool briefly before serving.

Macronutrients (estimated):

- Calories: 280 kcal
- Carbohydrates: 22 g
- Protein: 8 g
- Fat: 18 g

Boiled eggs and asparagus salad

Preparation time: 10 minutes

Cooking time: 10 minutes

Persons: 1

Ingredients:

- 2 large eggs
- 1/2 bunch asparagus, bottom end cut off
- 1 tablespoon olive oil
- 1 teaspoon Dijon mustard
- 1 tablespoon lemon juice
- Salt and pepper to taste
- Optional: a few radishes, cut into thin slices

Preparation:

1. **Boil the eggs:** Cook the eggs in a pan of boiling water for about 7-9 minutes for hard-boiled eggs. Then rinse under cold water, peel and set aside.
2. **Cook the asparagus:** Boil the asparagus in a separate pot of lightly salted water for about 3-5 minutes until tender but still firm to the bite. Rinse in ice water to stop the cooking and preserve the green color.
3. **Prepare the dressing:** In a small bowl, whisk together olive oil, Dijon mustard, lemon juice, salt and pepper to make the dressing.
4. **Serve the salad:** Place the cooled asparagus on a plate, halve or quarter the hard-boiled eggs and arrange on top of the asparagus. Optionally, you can now add the radish slices.
5. **Serve with dressing:** Drizzle the dressing over the salad and serve immediately.

Macronutrients (estimated):

- Calories: 275 kcal

- Carbohydrates: 9 g
- Protein: 13 g
- Fat: 20 g

Quark casserole with berries

Preparation time: 10 minutes
Cooking time: 25 minutes
Persons: 1
Ingredients:

- 1/2 cup low-fat quark
- 1 large egg
- 1/4 cup mixed berries (fresh or frozen)
- 1 tablespoon of honey or another sweetener of your choice
- 1/4 teaspoon vanilla extract
- Optional: A pinch of cinnamon

Preparation:

1. **Preheat the oven:** Preheat the oven to 180°C.
2. **Prepare the quark mixture:** In a medium bowl, thoroughly mix together the low-fat quark, egg, honey and vanilla extract. Optionally, you can add a pinch of cinnamon for extra flavor.
3. **Add the berries:** Carefully add the mixed berries to the quark mixture and mix gently so as not to crush the berries.
4. **Bake: Pour** the mixture into a small, ovenproof dish. Place the casserole in the preheated oven and bake for approx. 25 minutes until the surface is firm and golden in color.
5. **Serve:** Allow the casserole to cool briefly before serving. Optionally, you can garnish the casserole with additional fresh berries or a spoonful of honey.

Macronutrients (estimated):

- Calories: 270 kcal
- Carbohydrates: 21 g
- Protein: 22 g
- Fat: 6 g

Ratatouille with grilled chicken

Preparation time: 15 minutes
Cooking time: 30 minutes
Persons: 1
Ingredients:

- 1 small zucchini, cut into slices
- 1 small eggplant, cut into slices

- 1/2 red bell pepper, cut into strips
- 1/2 yellow bell pepper, cut into strips
- 1 tomato, diced
- 1 clove of garlic, finely chopped
- 150g chicken breast
- 1 tablespoon olive oil
- Salt and pepper to taste
- 1/2 teaspoon dried herbs (e.g. thyme, rosemary)
- Optional: fresh basil leaves for garnish

Preparation:

1. **Prepare the vegetables:** In a large bowl, mix the zucchini, eggplant, bell pepper, tomato and garlic with half the olive oil, salt, pepper and dried herbs.
2. **Cook the ratatouille:** Place the vegetables on a baking tray and bake in a preheated oven at 200°C for about 20-25 minutes until the vegetables are soft and slightly caramelized.
3. **Grill the chicken:** While the vegetables are in the oven, rub the chicken breast with the remaining olive oil, salt and pepper. Grill on a grill or in a grill pan for 5-7 minutes on each side until the chicken is cooked through.
4. **Leave the chicken to rest:** Remove the grilled chicken from the pan and leave to rest for a few minutes before slicing.
5. **Serve:** Place the ratatouille on a plate and arrange the grilled chicken breast on top. Optionally garnish with fresh basil leaves.

Macronutrients (estimated):

- Calories: 380 kcal
- Carbohydrates: 24 g
- Protein: 33 g
- Fat: 12 g

Beet salad with goat's cheese and walnuts

Preparation time: 10 minutes (if using pre-cooked beet)
Cooking time: 0 minutes
Persons: 1
Ingredients:

- 1 medium-sized beet, pre-cooked and sliced
- 30g goat's cheese, crumbled
- 1 tablespoon walnuts, roughly chopped
- 1 tablespoon olive oil
- 1/2 tablespoon balsamic vinegar
- Salt and pepper to taste
- A few leaves of fresh rocket or mixed salad

Preparation:

1. **Prepare the salad bed:** Spread the rocket or mixed salad on a plate as a base for the salad.
2. **Serve the beet:** Place the pre-cooked and sliced beet pieces on top of the salad.
3. **Add the goat's cheese and walnuts:** Sprinkle the crumbled goat's cheese and chopped walnuts over the beet.
4. **Prepare the dressing:** In a small bowl, mix the olive oil with the balsamic vinegar. Season with salt and pepper.
5. **Dress the salad:** Drizzle the dressing evenly over the salad.

Macronutrients (estimated):

- Calories: 260kcal
- Carbohydrates: 11 g
- Protein: 9 g
- Fat: 20 g

Spinach and feta pancakes (without flour)

Preparation time: 10 minutes
Cooking time: 10 minutes
Persons: 1
Ingredients:

- 2 large eggs
- 1/2 cup fresh spinach, finely chopped
- 30g feta cheese, crumbled
- 1 tablespoon of milk (or a dairy-free alternative)
- Salt and pepper to taste
- 1 teaspoon of olive oil for frying

Preparation:

1. **Whisk the eggs and milk:** In a bowl, whisk the eggs with the milk. Season with salt and pepper.
2. **Add the spinach and feta:** Add the finely chopped spinach and crumbled feta cheese to the egg mixture and mix well.
3. **Prepare the pancake mixture:** Heat the olive oil in a frying pan over a medium heat. Pour the pancake mixture into thc pan to form small pancakes.
4. **Fry the pancakes:** Let the pancakes fry for about 2-3 minutes on one side until they are firm, then carefully flip them over to fry the other side.
5. **Serve:** Place the finished spinach and feta pancakes on a plate and serve immediately.

Macronutrients (estimated):

- Calories: 250 kcal
- Carbohydrates: 4 g
- Protein: 16 g
- Fat: 20 g

Tuna salad with avocado and egg

Preparation time: 10 minutes
Cooking time: 10 minutes (if the egg is already cooked, the cooking time is omitted)
Persons: 1
Ingredients:

- 1 tin of tuna in its own juice (approx. 100g), drained
- 1 hard-boiled egg, chopped
- 1/2 ripe avocado, diced
- 1 tablespoon lemon juice
- 1 tablespoon olive oil
- Salt and pepper to taste
- Optional: a few leaves of fresh lettuce for the base

Preparation:

1. **Boil the egg:** If not already done, hard boil the egg, leave to cool, peel and chop.
2. **Prepare the tuna:** Place the drained tuna in a bowl.
3. **Add the avocado:** Dice the avocado and add to the tuna along with the chopped egg.
4. **Prepare the dressing:** Whisk together the lemon juice, olive oil, salt and pepper in a small bowl and pour over the tuna salad. Stir everything carefully so as not to mash the avocado.
5. **Serve:** Serve the tuna salad on a bed of fresh salad leaves or enjoy straight from the bowl.

Macronutrients (estimated):

- Calories: 365 kcal
- Carbohydrates: 6 g
- Protein: 26 g
- Fat: 27 g

Tomato and basil soup with mozzarella

Preparation time: 5 minutes
Cooking time: 20 minutes
Persons: 1
Ingredients:

- 2 large ripe tomatoes, diced
- 1/4 onion, finely chopped
- 1 clove of garlic, finely chopped
- 1 tablespoon olive oil
- 1/2 cup vegetable stock
- Fresh basil, a handful, roughly chopped
- 30g mozzarella, diced
- Salt and pepper to taste

Preparation:

1. **Sauté the onion and garlic:** Heat the olive oil in a saucepan and sauté the onion and garlic over a medium heat until soft.
2. **Add the tomatoes:** Add the diced tomatoes to the pot and cook for about 5 minutes until they soften.
3. **Cook the soup:** Add the vegetable stock and bring the soup to the boil. Then reduce the heat and simmer for about 10-15 minutes.
4. **Puree:** Remove the soup from the heat and puree with a hand blender or in a blender until smooth. Return to the pan, heat through and season to taste with salt and pepper.
5. **Serve with mozzarella and basil:** Pour the soup into a bowl, sprinkle with the mozzarella cubes and fresh basil and serve immediately.

Macronutrients (estimated):

- Calories: 222 kcal
- Carbohydrates: 12 g
- Protein: 8 g
- Fat: 16 g

Zucchini spaghetti with turkey bolognese

Preparation time: 10 minutes
Cooking time: 20 minutes
Persons: 1
Ingredients:

- 1 large zucchini, cut into a spiral to make spaghetti
- 150g minced turkey
- 1/2 tin of chopped tomatoes (approx. 200g)
- 1/4 onion, finely diced
- 1 clove of garlic, finely chopped
- 1 tablespoon olive oil
- Salt and pepper to taste
- 1 teaspoon dried oregano
- Optional: fresh basil to garnish

Preparation:

1. **Prepare the turkey bolognese:** Heat the olive oil in a frying pan over a medium heat. Add the onion and garlic and fry until soft. Add the turkey mince and fry until cooked through. Break the meat into small pieces.
2. **Add the tomatoes:** Add the chopped tomatoes, salt, pepper and oregano to the pan. Allow the sauce to simmer for about 10-15 minutes until it thickens.
3. **Cook the zucchini spaghetti: In the** meantime, bring water to the boil in another pan and blanch the zucchini spaghetti for approx. 1-2 minutes. Make sure that they do not become too soft. Then drain and leave to drain.

4. **To serve:** Place the zucchini spaghetti on a plate and spoon the turkey bolognese over it.
5. **Serve:** Garnish with fresh basil and serve immediately.

Macronutrients (estimated):

- Calories: 365 kcal
- Carbohydrates: 16 g
- Protein: 26 g
- Fat: 17 g

Zucchini soup with fresh ginger

Preparation time: 10 minutes
Cooking time: 20 minutes
Persons: 1
Ingredients:

- 1 large zucchini, roughly diced
- 1 small piece of fresh ginger (approx. 1 cm), finely chopped
- 1/2 onion, diced
- 1 clove of garlic, finely chopped
- 1 tablespoon olive oil
- 2 cups vegetable stock
- Salt and pepper to taste
- Optional: a squeeze of lemon juice

Preparation:

1. **Sauté the vegetables:** Heat the olive oil in a saucepan. Add the onion, garlic and ginger and fry over a medium heat until the onion softens.
2. **Add the zucchini: Add** the diced zucchini to the pan and fry for about 2-3 minutes.
3. **Cook:** Add the vegetable stock, bring to the boil and then reduce the heat. Leave the soup to simmer for about 15 minutes until the zucchini is soft.
4. **Puree:** Remove the soup from the heat and puree with a hand blender or in a blender until smooth. Season to taste with salt and pepper. Optionally, add a squeeze of lemon juice to lift the flavors.
5. **Serve:** Pour the soup into a bowl and serve hot.

Macronutrients (estimated):

- Calories: 170 kcal
- Carbohydrates: 16 g
- Protein: 4 g
- Fat: 8 g

Chapter 11: Recipes for dinner

Eggplant rolls with ricotta and spinach

Preparation time: 15 minutes
Cooking time: 25 minutes
Persons: 1
Ingredients:

- 1 large eggplant, cut into long, thin slices
- 1/2 cup ricotta
- 1 cup fresh spinach, roughly chopped
- 1 clove of garlic, finely chopped
- 1/4 cup grated Parmesan cheese
- 1/2 cup strained tomatoes
- Salt and pepper to taste
- 1 teaspoon olive oil

Preparation:

1. **Prepare the eggplant slices:** Sprinkle the eggplant slices with salt and leave to rest for about 10 minutes to reduce bitterness. Then rinse and pat dry.
2. **Spinach and ricotta filling:** In a bowl, mix together the ricotta, spinach, garlic, half the Parmesan, salt and pepper.
3. **Fill the eggplant rolls:** Place a tablespoon of the spinach and ricotta mixture on each slice of eggplant and roll up carefully.
4. **Bake:** Place the rolls in an ovenproof dish greased with olive oil, pour over the tomato purée and sprinkle with the remaining Parmesan. Bake at 180°C for about 20-25 minutes until the surface is golden brown.
5. **Serve:** Serve the eggplant rolls hot.

Macronutrients (estimated):

- Calories: approx. 320 kcal
- Carbohydrates: 22 g
- Protein: 17 g
- Fat: 16 g

Cauliflower steak with chimichurri sauce

Preparation time: 10 minutes
Cooking time: 20 minutes
Persons: 1
Ingredients:

- 2 thick slices of cauliflower (cut from the head as "steaks")

- 1 tablespoon olive oil
- Salt and pepper to taste

For the chimichurri sauce:

- 1/4 cup fresh parsley, finely chopped
- 1 clove of garlic, finely chopped
- 2 tablespoons olive oil
- 1 tablespoon red wine vinegar
- 1 teaspoon dried oregano
- A pinch of red pepper flakes
- Salt to taste

Preparation:

1. **Prepare the cauliflower:** Preheat the oven to 200°C. Brush the cauliflower slices with olive oil and season with salt and pepper. Place on a baking tray lined with baking paper.
2. **Bake:** Bake the cauliflower in the preheated oven for about 20 minutes until golden brown and soft, turning once.
3. **Mix the chimichurri sauce:** While the cauliflower is baking, mix all the ingredients for the chimichurri sauce in a small bowl. Season to taste and set aside.
4. **Finish the cauliflower steaks:** Remove the baked cauliflower steaks from the oven.
5. **Serve:** Arrange the cauliflower steaks on a plate and generously pour over the chimichurri sauce.

Macronutrients (estimated):

- Calories: 277 kcal
- Carbohydrates: 12 g
- Protein: 7 g
- Fat: 24 g

Creamy zucchini soup with chicken

Preparation time: 10 minutes
Cooking time: 20 minutes
Persons: 1
Ingredients:

- 1 large zucchini, diced
- 100g chicken breast, cooked and diced
- 1/2 onion, finely chopped
- 1 clove of garlic, finely chopped
- 1 cup chicken stock
- 1/4 cup light cream or coconut milk for a lactose-free option
- 1 tablespoon olive oil

- Salt and pepper to taste
- Fresh herbs for garnishing, e.g. parsley or basil

Preparation:

1. **Sauté the vegetables:** Heat the olive oil in a pan and sauté the onion and garlic until soft.
2. **Add the zucchini: Add** the diced zucchini to the pan and sauté for about 5 minutes until soft.
3. **Cook:** Add the chicken stock and bring to the boil. Reduce the heat and simmer the soup for about 10-15 minutes.
4. **Puree until creamy:** Remove the soup from the heat and puree with a hand blender or in a blender until smooth. Stir in the cream or coconut milk and season to taste with salt and pepper. Add the diced chicken breast and stir until warmed through in the soup.
5. **Serve:** Pour the soup into a bowl and garnish with fresh herbs.

Macronutrients (estimated):

- Calories: 320 kcal
- Carbohydrates: 17 g
- Protein: 27 g
- Fat: 16 g

Cod fillet in a bed of vegetables

Preparation time: 10 minutes
Cooking time: 20 minutes
Persons: 1
Ingredients:

- 1 cod fillet (approx. 150g)
- 1/2 zucchini, sliced
- 1/2 red bell pepper, cut into strips
- 1/2 yellow bell pepper, cut into strips
- 1/2 small red onion, cut into rings
- 2 tablespoons olive oil
- Salt and pepper to taste
- A few sprigs of fresh dill or parsley to garnish

Preparation:

1. **Preheat the oven:** Preheat the oven to 200°C.
2. **Prepare the vegetable bed:** Spread the vegetables (zucchini, bell pepper, onion) in an ovenproof dish, drizzle with half the olive oil, season with salt and pepper and mix well.
3. **Prepare the cod:** Season the cod fillet with salt and pepper, drizzle with the remaining olive oil and place on the bed of vegetables.
4. **Bake:** Bake the vegetables and fish in the preheated oven for about 20 minutes, or until the fish is cooked

through and the vegetables are tender.

5. **Serve:** Place the cod fillet in a bed of vegetables on a plate and garnish with fresh dill or parsley.

Macronutrients (estimated):

- Calories: 365 kcal
- Carbohydrates: 12 g
- Protein: 27 g
- Fat: 16 g

Protein-rich lentil and tomato soup

Preparation time: 5 minutes
Cooking time: 25 minutes
Persons: 1
Ingredients:

- 1/2 cup red lentils
- 1/2 tin of chopped tomatoes (approx. 200g)
- 1/4 onion, finely diced
- 1 clove of garlic, finely chopped
- 1/2 carrot, diced
- 2 cups vegetable stock
- 1 teaspoon olive oil
- Salt and pepper to taste
- 1/2 teaspoon dried oregano or basil

Preparation:

1. **Sauté the vegetables:** Heat the olive oil in a medium saucepan. Add the onion, garlic and carrot and sauté over a medium heat until the onion is translucent.
2. **Add the lentils and tomatoes:** Add the red lentils and chopped tomatoes to the pot and stir well.
3. **Cook:** Add the vegetable stock, bring to the boil and then reduce the heat. Season with salt, pepper and oregano or basil. Simmer for about 20 minutes until the lentils are soft.
4. **Season to taste:** Taste the soup and season with more salt and pepper if necessary.
5. **Serve:** Pour the finished soup into a bowl and serve hot.

Macronutrients (estimated):

- Calories: 340 kcal
- Carbohydrates: 42 g
- Protein: 19 g
- Fat: 6 g

Lamb's lettuce with grilled salmon

Preparation time: 5 minutes

Cooking time: 10 minutes

Persons: 1

Ingredients:

- 150g salmon fillet
- 2 cups lamb's lettuce, washed and dried
- 1/2 small red onion, cut into thin rings
- 1/2 avocado, diced
- 1 tablespoon of olive oil (for the salmon)
- 1 teaspoon of olive oil (for the salad)
- 1 tablespoon balsamic vinegar
- Salt and pepper to taste
- Optional: A few chopped walnuts or almonds for extra texture

Preparation:

1. **Prepare the salmon:** Season the salmon with salt and pepper and brush with 1 tablespoon of olive oil.
2. **Grill the salmon:** Grill the salmon over a medium heat on a grill or in a grill pan for 4-5 minutes on each side until cooked through but still juicy.
3. **Dress the salad:** In a large bowl, mix the lamb's lettuce with the red onion and diced avocado. Dress with 1 teaspoon of olive oil and balsamic vinegar. Season to taste with salt and pepper.
4. **Cut up the salmon:** Cut the grilled salmon into large pieces or leave whole, depending on your preference.
5. **Serve:** Place the dressed lamb's lettuce on a plate, arrange the grilled salmon on top and optionally sprinkle with chopped walnuts or almonds.

Macronutrients (estimated):

- Calories: 420 kcal
- Carbohydrates: 9 g
- Protein: 27 g
- Fat: 33 g

Roast chicken with broccoli and almonds

Preparation time: 10 minutes

Cooking time: 20 minutes

Persons: 1

Ingredients:

- 150g chicken breast
- 1 cup broccoli florets
- 2 tablespoons slivered almonds
- 1 tablespoon olive oil

- Salt and pepper to taste
- 1/2 teaspoon paprika powder
- Optional: lemon juice for drizzling

Preparation:

1. **Prepare the chicken:** Season the chicken breast with salt, pepper and paprika powder.
2. **Fry the chicken:** Heat the olive oil in a frying pan and fry the chicken breast for 5-7 minutes on each side until cooked through. Then remove from the pan and set aside.
3. **Cook the broccoli:** Sauté the broccoli florets in the same oil for about 5 minutes until they are al dente. Season with salt and pepper.
4. **Toast the almonds:** Lightly toast the almond slivers in a separate pan without oil until they are golden brown.
5. **To serve:** Arrange the roasted chicken with the broccoli on a plate, sprinkle with the toasted almonds and optionally drizzle with a little lemon juice.

Macronutrients (estimated):

- Calories: 420 kcal
- Carbohydrates: 12 g
- Protein: 33 g
- Fat: 22 g

Chicken breast with ratatouille

Preparation time: 15 minutes
Cooking time: 30 minutes
Persons: 1
Ingredients:

- 1 chicken breast (approx. 150g)
- 1/4 zucchini, cut into cubes
- 1/4 eggplant, cut into cubes
- 1/4 red bell pepper, cut into cubes
- 1/4 yellow bell pepper, cut into cubes
- 1 small tomato, diced
- 1 small onion, finely diced
- 1 clove of garlic, finely chopped
- 2 tablespoons olive oil
- Salt and pepper to taste
- 1/2 teaspoon dried herbs (e.g. thyme, rosemary)

Preparation:

1. **Prepare the chicken breast:** Season the chicken breast with salt and pepper and fry in 1 tablespoon of olive oil for 5-7 minutes on each side until cooked through. Remove from the pan and keep warm.

2. **Sauté the vegetables:** Heat the remaining olive oil in the same pan. Add the onion and garlic and sauté for 2-3 minutes.
3. **Prepare the ratatouille:** Add the zucchini, eggplant, bell pepper and tomato, season with salt, pepper and dried herbs. Simmer over a medium heat for about 20 minutes until the vegetables are soft.
4. **Season the vegetables to taste:** Check whether the ratatouille needs any more seasoning and season if necessary.
5. **Serve:** Place the ratatouille on a plate and arrange the chicken breast on top.

Macronutrients (estimated):

- Calories: 365 kcal
- Carbohydrates: 16 g
- Protein: 33 g
- Fat: 16 g

Ginger and carrot soup with coconut milk

Preparation time: 10 minutes
Cooking time: 20 minutes
Persons: 1
Ingredients:

- 200g carrots, peeled and roughly chopped
- 1/2 small onion, diced
- 1 cm fresh ginger, peeled and finely chopped
- 1/2 tin of coconut milk (approx. 200 ml)
- 1 cup vegetable stock
- 1 teaspoon olive oil
- Salt and pepper to taste
- Optional: A squeeze of lemon juice or lime juice for extra freshness

Preparation:

1. **Sauté the vegetables:** Heat the olive oil in a pan and fry the onion and ginger over a medium heat until the onion is translucent.
2. **Add the carrots:** Add the carrot pieces to the pan and fry for a few minutes.
3. **Cook:** Add the vegetable stock, bring to the boil and then reduce the heat. Simmer for about 15-20 minutes until the carrots are soft.
4. **Puree and add the coconut milk:** Remove the soup from the heat and puree with a hand blender until smooth. Stir in the coconut milk, season to taste with salt and pepper and reheat if necessary.
5. **Serve:** Pour the soup into a bowl, refine with an optional squeeze of lemon or lime juice and serve.

Macronutrients (estimated):

- Calories: 330 kcal

- Carbohydrates: 22 g
- Protein: 6 g
- Fat: 16 g

Scallops on a bed of spinach with lemon sauce

Preparation time: 10 minutes
Cooking time: 10 minutes
Persons: 1
Ingredients:

- 4 large scallops
- 2 cups fresh spinach
- 1 tablespoon olive oil
- 1 clove of garlic, finely chopped
- Juice and zest of 1/2 lemon
- Salt and pepper to taste
- Optional: a few pine nuts to garnish

Preparation:

1. **Prepare the scallops:** Pat the scallops dry and season with salt and pepper. Heat the olive oil in a frying pan over a medium heat and sear the scallops for 2-3 minutes on each side until they have a golden brown crust. Remove from the pan and set aside.
2. **Prepare the spinach:** Briefly fry the garlic in the same oil, add the spinach and sauté for 2-3 minutes until it collapses. Season with salt and pepper.
3. **Make the lemon sauce:** Deglaze the pan juices with the lemon juice and zest and bring to the boil briefly to combine the flavors.
4. **To serve:** Arrange the spinach as a bed on a plate, place the scallops on top and pour over the lemon sauce.
5. **Serve:** Optionally garnish with some toasted pine nuts and serve immediately.

Macronutrients (estimated):

- Calories: 260 kcal
- Carbohydrates: 5 g
- Protein: 25 g
- Fat: 16 g

Boiled eggs and asparagus salad

Preparation time: 10 minutes
Cooking time: 10 minutes
Persons: 1
Ingredients:

- 2 large eggs

- 1 bunch of green asparagus, bottom third removed
- 1 teaspoon olive oil
- Salt and pepper to taste
- 1/2 lemon, juice
- 1 tablespoon of roasted pine nuts or almonds
- Optional: A few leaves of fresh basil or parsley

Preparation:

1. **Boil the eggs:** Bring the eggs to the boil in a pan of water and cook for approx. 7-9 minutes for hard-boiled eggs. Then rinse, peel and cut in half or quarters.
2. **Prepare the asparagus:** Blanch the green asparagus in a grill pan or in a pot of boiling salted water for 2-3 minutes until it is al dente. Then quench in ice water to stop the cooking and preserve the green color.
3. **Dress the salad:** Place the cooled asparagus in a salad bowl, dress with olive oil, lemon juice, salt and pepper.
4. **To serve:** Arrange the dressed asparagus on a plate, place the boiled eggs on top and sprinkle with toasted pine nuts or almonds.
5. **Serve:** Optionally garnish with fresh herbs such as basil or parsley and serve immediately.

Macronutrients (estimated):

- Calories: 300 kcal
- Carbohydrates: 9 g
- Protein: 17 g
- Fat: 19 g

Salmon fillet with green asparagus and quinoa

Preparation time: 10 minutes
Cooking time: 20 minutes
Persons: 1
Ingredients:

- 1 salmon fillet (approx. 150g)
- 1 cup green asparagus, bottom third removed
- 1/2 cup quinoa
- 1 teaspoon olive oil
- Salt and pepper to taste
- 1 lemon slice for garnish
- Optional: A few sprigs of fresh dill or parsley

Preparation:

1. **Cook the quinoa: Cook the** quinoa in a pan of water according to the packet instructions until it is soft and fluffy, usually about 15 minutes. Then drain and set aside.
2. **Fry the salmon:** Season the salmon fillet with salt and pepper. Heat the olive oil in a pan and fry the salmon

for 3-4 minutes on each side until cooked through.

3. **Prepare the asparagus:** While the salmon is frying, cook the green asparagus in another pan or pot with a little water or steam for 3-5 minutes until it is al dente.
4. **To serve:** Place the quinoa on a plate and arrange the fried salmon and green asparagus next to it.
5. **Serve:** Garnish the dish with a slice of lemon and optionally sprinkle with fresh dill or parsley.

Macronutrients (estimated):

- Calories: 440 kcal
- Carbohydrates: 33 g
- Protein: 26 g
- Fat: 16 g

Mediterranean vegetable casserole

Preparation time: 15 minutes

Cooking time: 25 minutes

Persons: 1

Ingredients:

- 1/2 zucchini, sliced
- 1/2 eggplant, sliced
- 1 tomato, sliced
- 1/4 red bell pepper, cut into strips
- 1/4 yellow bell pepper, cut into strips
- 1 small onion, cut into rings
- 1 clove of garlic, finely chopped
- 2 tablespoons of strained tomatoes
- 1 teaspoon olive oil
- Salt and pepper to taste
- 1/2 teaspoon dried oregano
- 30g feta cheese, crumbled

Preparation:

1. **Prepare the vegetables:** Cut the zucchini, eggplant, tomato, red and yellow peppers and onion into slices or strips.
2. **Layer the vegetables:** In a small casserole dish, first place a layer of strained tomatoes, then alternate layers of vegetable slices. Sprinkle a little garlic between the layers and season with salt, pepper and oregano.
3. **Sprinkle with cheese:** Sprinkle the crumbled feta cheese over the vegetables.
4. **Bake:** Bake the casserole in a preheated oven at 180°C for about 25 minutes until the vegetables are soft and the cheese is lightly browned.
5. **Serve:** Serve the Mediterranean vegetable casserole hot from the oven.

Macronutrients (estimated):

- Calories: 260 kcal
- Carbohydrates: 22 g
- Protein: 15 g
- Fat: 17 g

Low-calorie turkey goulash with peppers

Preparation time: 10 minutes
Cooking time: 30 minutes
Persons: 1
Ingredients:

- 150g turkey breast, cut into cubes
- 1 red bell pepper, cut into strips
- 1 green bell pepper, cut into strips
- 1/2 onion, finely diced
- 1 clove of garlic, finely chopped
- 1 tin of chopped tomatoes (approx. 200g)
- 1 teaspoon paprika powder
- 1/2 teaspoon ground caraway seeds
- 1 tablespoon olive oil
- Salt and pepper to taste
- Optional: Fresh parsley to garnish

Preparation:

1. **Brown the turkey:** Heat the olive oil in a pan and sear the turkey cubes on all sides until lightly browned. Remove from the pan and set aside.
2. **Sauté the vegetables:** Sauté the onion and garlic in the same pan until soft. Add the bell pepper strips and sauté for a few minutes.
3. **Assemble the goulash:** Return the browned turkey cubes to the pan. Add the chopped tomatoes, paprika powder and caraway seeds. Season with salt and pepper and stir well.
4. **Cook:** Simmer the goulash over a low heat for about 20-25 minutes until the turkey cubes are tender and the sauce has thickened.
5. **Serve:** Arrange the turkey goulash on a plate and optionally garnish with fresh parsley.

Macronutrients (estimated):

- Calories: 330 kcal
- Carbohydrates: 16 g
- Protein: 31 g
- Fat: 14 g

Oven vegetables with tofu and sesame seeds

Preparation time: 10 minutes

Cooking time: 25 minutes
Persons: 1
Ingredients:

- 200g firm tofu, cut into cubes
- 1/2 zucchini, cut into half moons
- 1/2 red bell pepper, cut into strips
- 1/2 yellow bell pepper, cut into strips
- 1/2 small red onion, cut into wedges
- 1 tablespoon olive oil
- 1 teaspoon sesame seeds
- Salt and pepper to taste
- 1/2 teaspoon paprika powder
- Optional: A splash of soy sauce for extra flavor

Preparation:

1. **Preheat the oven:** Preheat the oven to 200°C.
2. **Prepare the vegetables and tofu:** Mix the tofu and vegetables in a large bowl with olive oil, salt, pepper and paprika until everything is evenly coated.
3. **Bake:** Spread the tofu and vegetable mixture on a baking tray lined with baking paper and bake in the preheated oven for about 20-25 minutes, until the vegetables are soft and the tofu is slightly crispy around the edges.
4. **Sprinkle with sesame seeds:** Remove the baked vegetables and tofu from the oven and sprinkle with sesame seeds. Optionally, add a splash of soy sauce over the finished dish.
5. **Serve:** Serve the baked vegetables with tofu and sesame seeds immediately.

Macronutrients (estimated):

- Calories: 360 kcal
- Carbohydrates: 16 g
- Protein: 22 g
- Fat: 16 g

Peppers stuffed with quinoa and vegetables

Preparation time: 15 minutes
Cooking time: 25 minutes
Persons: 1
Ingredients:

- 1 large bell bell pepper
- 1/4 cup quinoa
- 1/2 cup vegetable stock
- 1/4 zucchini, diced

- 1/4 red onion, finely diced
- 1 small carrot, diced
- 1 clove of garlic, finely chopped
- 1 tablespoon olive oil
- Salt and pepper to taste
- 1 teaspoon dried oregano
- 2 tablespoons grated cheese (optional)

Preparation:

1. **Cook the quinoa:** Cook the quinoa in the vegetable stock according to the packet instructions until soft and the liquid has been absorbed.
2. **Prepare the vegetables:** While the quinoa is cooking, heat the olive oil in a pan and sauté the onion, carrot, zucchini and garlic until the vegetables are soft. Season with salt, pepper and oregano.
3. **Prepare the peppers:** Cut the bell pepper in half and remove the seeds. Stuff the quinoa and vegetable mixture into the bell pepper halves.
4. **Bake:** Place the stuffed bell pepper halves in an ovenproof dish and bake in a preheated oven at 180°C for about 20 minutes. Optionally, sprinkle with grated cheese in the last 5 minutes.
5. **Serve:** Remove the stuffed peppers from the oven and serve warm.

Macronutrients (estimated):

- Calories: 360 kcal
- Carbohydrates: 44 g
- Protein: 14 g
- Fat: 16 g

Quark casserole with berries

Preparation time: 10 minutes
Cooking time: 20 minutes
Persons: 1
Ingredients:

- 150g low-fat quark
- 1/2 cup mixed berries (fresh or frozen)
- 1 egg
- 1 tablespoon of honey or another sweetener of your choice
- 1 teaspoon vanilla extract
- 2 tablespoons oat flakes
- A pinch of cinnamon
- Optional: A few flaked almonds for decoration

Preparation:

1. **Preheat the oven:** Preheat the oven to 180°C.
2. **Prepare the mixture:** In a bowl, thoroughly mix the low-fat quark, egg, honey and vanilla extract. Add the rolled oats and cinnamon and mix well.
3. **Add the berries:** Carefully fold the berries into the quark mixture. If using frozen berries, do not defrost them beforehand.
4. **Bake:** Pour the mixture into a small baking dish lined with baking paper or greased. Optionally, sprinkle with flaked almonds. Bake in the preheated oven for about 20 minutes until the casserole is firm and lightly golden brown.
5. **Serve:** Remove the quark casserole from the oven and leave to cool slightly. Serve warm or cold.

Macronutrients (estimated):

- Calories: 330 kcal
- Carbohydrates: 35 g
- Protein: 22 g
- Fat: 8 g

Beef fillet strips on rocket salad

Preparation time: 10 minutes
Cooking time: 10 minutes
Persons: 1
Ingredients:

- 150g fillet of beef, cut into strips
- 2 cups rocket
- 1/2 red bell pepper, cut into thin strips
- 1/4 cucumber, cut into thin slices
- 1 tablespoon of olive oil (for the meat)
- 1 teaspoon balsamic vinegar
- 1 teaspoon of olive oil (for the salad)
- Salt and pepper to taste
- Optional: Parmesan shavings for garnish

Preparation:

1. **Brown the fillet of beef:** Season the fillet of beef with salt and pepper. Heat 1 tablespoon of olive oil in a pan and sear the beef fillet strips over a high heat for approx. 2-3 minutes on each side until they have reached the desired doneness. Remove from the pan and set aside.
2. **Prepare the salad:** Mix the rocket, red bell pepper and cucumber slices in a bowl.
3. **Mix the salad dressing:** Mix the balsamic vinegar with 1 teaspoon of olive oil and season with salt and pepper. Pour the dressing over the salad and mix well.
4. **To serve:** Arrange the rocket salad on a plate and arrange the warm beef fillet strips on top.
5. **Serve:** Optionally garnish with Parmesan shavings and serve immediately.

Macronutrients (estimated):

- Calories: 333 kcal
- Carbohydrates: 9 g
- Protein: 26 g
- Fat: 18 g

Spinach and feta omelette without flour

Preparation time: 5 minutes
Cooking time: 10 minutes
Persons: 1
Ingredients:

- 2 large eggs
- 1 cup fresh s
- spinach, coarsely chopped
- 30g feta cheese, crumbled
- 1 tablespoon olive oil
- Salt and pepper to taste
- Optional: a pinch of nutmeg or paprika powder for extra flavor

Preparation:

1. **Beat the eggs:** Beat the eggs in a bowl and season with salt and pepper. Optionally, add a pinch of nutmeg or paprika powder.
2. **Prepare the spinach:** Heat the olive oil in a pan and briefly sauté the spinach until it collapses. Remove from the pan and set aside.
3. **Prepare the omelette:** In the same pan, pour the beaten eggs over a medium heat and spread evenly. Pour the steamed spinach and feta cheese crumbs over one half of the omelette.
4. **Fold the omelette:** Once the eggs have set but the top is still slightly moist, fold the omelette over to seal the filling.
5. **Serve:** Slide the omelette onto a plate and serve immediately.

Macronutrients (estimated):

- Calories: 340 kcal
- Carbohydrates: 3 g
- Protein: 20 g
- Fat: 25 g

Tuna steak with Mediterranean vegetables

Preparation time: 10 minutes
Cooking time: 20 minutes
Persons: 1

Ingredients:

- 1 tuna steak (approx. 150g)
- 1/2 zucchini, sliced
- 1/2 eggplant, sliced
- 1 small red bell pepper, cut into strips
- 1 small yellow bell pepper, cut into strips
- 10 cherry tomatoes, halved
- 2 tablespoons olive oil
- Salt and pepper to taste
- 1 teaspoon dried oregano
- 1 clove of garlic, finely chopped
- Fresh lemon juice for drizzling

Preparation:

1. **Prepare the vegetables:** Place the zucchini, eggplant, red and yellow peppers and cherry tomatoes in a bowl, mix with 1 tablespoon of olive oil, salt, pepper, oregano and garlic.
2. **Bake the vegetables:** Spread the vegetables on a baking tray lined with baking paper and bake at 200°C for approx. 15-20 minutes until soft and lightly browned.
3. **Fry the tuna steak:** Season the tuna steak with salt and pepper. Heat the remaining tablespoon of olive oil in a pan and fry the tuna steak for approx. 2-3 minutes on each side (depending on the desired degree of doneness).
4. **Leave the tuna steak to rest:** Remove the tuna steak from the pan and leave to rest briefly.
5. **Serve:** Arrange the baked Mediterranean vegetables on a plate, place the tuna steak on top and drizzle with fresh lemon juice.

Macronutrients (estimated):

- Calories: 440 kcal
- Carbohydrates: 24 g
- Protein: 32 g
- Fat: 22 g

Baked cauliflower with parmesan

Preparation time: 10 minutes

Cooking time: 20 minutes

Persons: 1

Ingredients:

- 1/2 head of cauliflower, divided into florets
- 2 tablespoons olive oil
- Salt and pepper to taste
- 1/4 cup grated Parmesan cheese
- 1 teaspoon Italian herbs (optional)

- 1 clove of garlic, finely chopped (optional)

Preparation:

1. **Prepare the cauliflower:** Mix the cauliflower florets well with the olive oil, salt, pepper, (optional) garlic and Italian herbs in a bowl.
2. **Bake:** Spread the cauliflower florets on a baking tray lined with baking paper and bake at 200°C for approx. 15-20 minutes until soft and lightly browned around the edges.
3. **Sprinkle with cheese:** Sprinkle the grated Parmesan cheese over the cauliflower florets and bake for a further 5 minutes until the cheese has melted and is lightly golden brown.
4. **Finish off:** Remove the baked cauliflower from the oven and leave to cool briefly.
5. **Serve:** Arrange the baked cauliflower on a plate and serve immediately.

Macronutrients (estimated):

- Calories: 270 kcal
- Carbohydrates: 12 g
- Protein: 15 g
- Fat: 19 g

Vegetarian zucchini lasagne

Preparation time: 15 minutes
Cooking time: 30 minutes
Persons: 1
Ingredients:

- 1 large zucchini, cut lengthwise into thin slices
- 1/2 cup strained tomatoes
- 1/4 cup ricotta
- 1/4 cup grated mozzarella
- 1 tablespoon grated Parmesan cheese
- 1/2 small onion, finely diced
- 1 clove of garlic, finely chopped
- 1 teaspoon olive oil
- Salt and pepper to taste
- 1/2 teaspoon dried oregano
- Fresh basil leaves for garnish

Preparation:

1. **Prepare the zucchinis:** Cut the zucchinis into long, thin slices using a vegetable peeler or mandoline slicer. Salt lightly and set aside for 10 minutes to remove excess liquid.
2. **Prepare the tomato sauce:** Heat the olive oil in a pan, sauté the onion and garlic. Add the strained tomatoes, season with salt, pepper and oregano and simmer for approx. 10 minutes.

3. **Layer the lasagne:** Lightly grease a small oven dish. Lay out a layer of zucchini slices, spread some tomato sauce on top, followed by a spoonful of ricotta. Repeat the process until all the ingredients have been used and finish with a layer of mozzarella.
4. **Bake:** Bake at 180°C for about 20 minutes until the cheese is golden brown and the zucchini is soft. Sprinkle over the Parmesan in the last few minutes.
5. **Serve:** Leave the lasagne to cool briefly and garnish with fresh basil leaves before serving.

Macronutrients (estimated):

- Calories: 320 kcal
- Carbohydrates: 18 g
- Protein: 19 g
- Fat: 17 g

Spicy pumpkin stew with chicken

Preparation time: 15 minutes
Cooking time: 30 minutes
Persons: 1
Ingredients:

- 150g chicken breast, cut into cubes
- 1 cup pumpkin, diced
- 1/2 tin of chopped tomatoes (approx. 200g)
- 1/2 onion, finely diced
- 1 clove of garlic, finely chopped
- 1/2 red bell pepper, diced
- 1/2 cup chicken stock
- 1 teaspoon olive oil
- 1/4 teaspoon chili powder (or to taste)
- 1/4 teaspoon cumin
- Salt and pepper to taste
- Fresh coriander to garnish

Preparation:

1. **Fry the chicken:** Heat the olive oil in a pan and fry the chicken breast cubes on all sides until lightly browned. Remove from the pan and set aside.
2. **Sauté the vegetables:** In the same pot, saute onion, garlic and red bell bell pepper over medium heat until soft.
3. **Assemble the stew:** Add the diced pumpkin, chopped tomatoes and chicken stock to the vegetables. Add the chili powder, cumin, salt and pepper and stir.
4. **Cook:** Return the chicken cubes to the pan. Bring everything to the boil, then reduce the heat and simmer with the lid on for about 20-25 minutes until the pumpkin is soft and the chicken is cooked through.
5. **Serve:** Place the stew in a bowl and garnish with fresh coriander.

Macronutrients (estimated):

- Calories: 380 kcal
- Carbohydrates: 29 g
- Protein: 31 g
- Fat: 14 g

Pike-perch fillet on a bed of lentils

Preparation time: 15 minutes
Cooking time: 25 minutes
Persons: 1
Ingredients:

- 1 zander fillet (approx. 150g)
- 1/2 cup green lentils
- 1 small carrot, finely diced
- 1/2 small onion, finely diced
- 1 clove of garlic, finely chopped
- 1 tablespoon olive oil
- 1 cup vegetable stock
- Salt and pepper to taste
- Fresh herbs (e.g. parsley or dill) to garnish

Preparation:

1. **Cook the lentils:** Wash the lentils thoroughly and bring to the boil in a pan with twice the amount of vegetable stock. Simmer on a low heat for about 20 minutes until they are soft but still have a bite. If necessary, add more stock during cooking.
2. **Sauté the vegetables:** While the lentils are cooking, heat the olive oil in another pan and sauté the onion, carrot and garlic over a medium heat until soft.
3. **Prepare the zander fillet:** Season the zander fillet with salt and pepper. Heat a little olive oil in a separate pan and fry the fillet on the skin side for approx. 3-4 minutes, then turn and finish cooking on the other side for 2 minutes.
4. **Serve the lentils:** Mix the cooked lentils with the sautéed vegetables and place on a plate. Season to taste with salt and pepper.
5. **Serve:** Arrange the pike-perch fillet on the bed of lentils and garnish with fresh herbs.

Macronutrients (estimated):

- Calories: 480 kcal
- Carbohydrates: 37 g
- Protein: 33 g
- Fat: 14 g

Zucchini pasta with avocado pesto

Preparation time: 10 minutes
Cooking time: 0 minutes (raw)
Persons: 1
Ingredients:

- 1 large zucchini
- 1/2 ripe avocado
- 1 garlic clove
- A handful of fresh basil
- 1 tablespoon pine nuts (optionally roasted for more flavor)
- 2 tablespoons olive oil
- Juice of 1/2 lemon
- Salt and pepper to taste
- Parmesan cheese or yeast flakes for garnish (optional)

Preparation:

1. **Prepare the zucchinis:** Use a spiral cutter or vegetable peeler to shape the zucchinis into noodles. No further steps required for raw zucchini noodles. Optionally, the zucchini noodles can be blanched in boiling water for 1-2 minutes if a softer consistency is desired.
2. **Prepare the pesto:** Place the avocado, garlic, basil, pine nuts, olive oil and lemon juice in a blender. Puree everything to a smooth pesto. Season to taste with salt and pepper.
3. **Mix the zucchini noodles: Place** the zucchini noodles in a bowl and add the avocado pesto on top. Mix everything well so that the pasta is evenly coated with the pesto.
4. **To serve:** Serve the zucchini noodles with avocado pesto on a plate.
5. **Serve:** Optionally garnish with Parmesan cheese or yeast flakes and fresh basil.

Macronutrients (estimated):

- Calories: 390 kcal
- Carbohydrates: 18 g
- Protein: 9 g
- Fat: 33 g

Chapter 9: Success stories

In this chapter, we dive into the moving and inspiring stories of people who have experienced extraordinary transformations with the help of Dr. Nowzaradan's diet plan. These success stories serve as vivid examples that with determination, hard work and the right guidance, remarkable change is possible.

Emilia's decision to start a new life

Emilia, a 40-year-old single mother, was faced with the challenge of transforming her life after her weight caused serious health problems. With a starting point of over 150 kilograms and the goal of being a more active role model for her daughter, she followed Dr. Nowzaradan's diet plan with a mixture of determination and hope. Over the course of a year, with strict adherence to the diet and a gradually increased exercise program, Emilia lost an impressive 70 kilograms. Her story is a testament to how a mother turned her love and concern for her family into the power to change.

Tom's struggle and triumph

Tom, a 55-year-old former firefighter, was facing retirement overshadowed by obesity and related health issues. After years of looking after the wellbeing of others, he decided it was time to look after his own health. With a strict diet plan and the support of Dr. Nowzaradan, Tom began his weight loss journey. By changing his eating habits and walking every day, he lost 60 kilograms within 18 months and found a new, healthier lifestyle.

Lisa's path to self-discovery

Lisa, a 32-year-old graphic designer, suffered from low self-esteem and social isolation due to her weight. Her decision to follow Dr. Nowzaradan's diet was less about losing weight and more about rediscovering her true self. Through a combination of nutritional dieting, regular yoga and meditation, Lisa transformed not only her body, but also her mind and emotional well-being. Within a year, she lost 40 kilograms and gained a new perspective on life and her own possibilities.

The meaning behind the stories

These stories demonstrate not only the physical transformations possible through Dr. Nowzaradan's diet plan, but also the deep emotional and psychological development that takes place during the process. Each person has overcome their own challenges and struggles, learning valuable lessons about themselves, about resilience, and about the power of change.

Chapter 10: Frequently asked questions (FAQs)

1. can I go vegetarian or vegan on Dr. Nowzaradan's diet?

Yes, it is possible to follow Dr. Nowzaradan's diet principles even as a vegetarian or vegan. The focus is on low calorie intake with high nutritional value, which can be easily achieved through plant-based foods. Be sure to include a variety of protein sources such as legumes, tofu, tempeh and whole grains, and meet your vitamin and mineral needs with a wide range of fruits and vegetables.

2. how can I avoid food cravings?

Cravings can be minimized by eating regular meals and snacks that are rich in protein and fibre. These nutrients ensure a longer-lasting feeling of fullness. Also drink plenty of water, as thirst is often misinterpreted as hunger. Also identify emotional triggers for cravings and develop alternative coping strategies.

3. how often should I exercise during Dr. Nowzaradan's diet?

The recommendation varies depending on individual fitness and state of health. A good starting point is moderate exercise of at least 150 minutes per week. This can include walking, swimming, cycling or any other activity that you enjoy and can do regularly. The important thing is to start slowly and gradually increase the intensity.

4 What do I do if my weight loss comes to a standstill?

Weight plateaus are a normal part of the weight loss process. Start by reviewing your calorie intake and make sure you continue to stick to your diet plan. Also review your exercise routine - it may be time to change the intensity or type of exercise. Patience and consistency are key to success here.

5 Is it safe to follow Dr. Nowzaradan's diet without medical supervision?

Although Dr. Nowzaradan's diet principles are focused on healthy eating and weight loss, it is advisable to seek medical advice before starting any diet or new exercise program, especially if you have pre-existing medical conditions or are taking medication.

6. how can I ensure that I maintain my weight after the diet?

Maintaining your weight after dieting requires a lifelong commitment to healthy eating habits and regular physical activity. Continue the principles of eating a balanced diet, watching your portion sizes and staying active. It is also helpful to conduct regular self-checks and make adjustments as needed.

7. how do I deal with social occasions where unhealthy food is offered?

Plan ahead and eat a small, nutritious meal before going to social events to avoid overeating. At events, consciously choose healthier options and control your portion sizes. Allow yourself occasional small indulgences to avoid feeling deprived and then return to your healthy habits.

8. can I drink alcohol while following Dr. Nowzaradan's diet?

While moderate alcohol consumption may be fine for most people, it's important to note that alcohol adds extra calories that can hinder your weight loss. Alcohol can also weaken your resolve to stick to healthy eating habits. If you choose to drink alcohol, do so in moderation and choose drinks with lower calorie content.

9. how do I deal with the feeling of hunger when I eat fewer calories?

To minimize hunger pangs, focus on high-volume, nutrient-dense foods that are rich in fiber and protein, as these will keep you feeling fuller for longer. Vegetables, fruit, whole grains and lean protein can help you feel fuller without exceeding your calorie intake. It's also important to drink enough water, as dehydration can often be misinterpreted as hunger.

10. how can I eat out without interrupting my diet?

When eating out, check the menu in advance and plan your meal accordingly. Ask for healthier cooking methods such as grilling or steaming and ask for sauces or dressings to be served separately. Focus on dishes that consist mainly of vegetables and lean proteins and pay attention to portion sizes.

11. how important is it to drink water during the diet?

Drinking water is crucial during any diet as it not only helps to keep the body hydrated, but also promotes satiety and can help to reduce overall calorie consumption. Experts recommend drinking at least 8 glasses of water a day, or more if you are active or live in a hot climate.

12. what should I do if I have a relapse and eat unhealthy food?

A relapse is not the end of your journey, but part of the learning process. It is important not to judge yourself too harshly and instead reflect on what led to the relapse in order to better manage similar situations in the future. Focus on getting back to your healthy habits and use the experience to strengthen your resolve.

13. how do I find the right balance between pleasure and healthy eating?

A balanced diet means eating a predominantly healthy diet, but also allowing yourself occasional indulgences. The key lies in moderate indulgence and mindfulness when eating. Allow yourself small amounts of your favorite foods without losing control and consciously enjoy each meal.

Download your FREE BONUS by scanning the QR code.
No e-mail is required.

Thank you for your purchase.
I would be very pleased if you would leave an honest review on Amazon.

www.ingramcontent.com/pod-product-compliance
Ingram Content Group UK Ltd.
Pitfield, Milton Keynes, MK11 3LW, UK
UKHW050637170725
6942UKWH00020B/169

9 798224 013623